Ben Stacy Jerrik (Ed.)

Spinal Muscular Atrophy Type 2

AF525401

Ben Stacy Jerrik (Ed.)

Spinal Muscular Atrophy Type 2

Atrophy, Autosomal, Recessive, Disease, Spinal, Medicine

Part Press

Imprint

Permission is granted to copy, distribute and/or modify this document under the terms of the GNU Free Documentation License, Version 1.2 or any later version published by the Free Software Foundation; with no Invariant Sections, with the Front-Cover Texts, and with the Back- Cover Texts. A copy of the license is included in the section entitled "GNU Free Documentation License".

All parts of this book are extracted from Wikipedia, the free encyclopedia (www.wikipedia.org).

You can get detailed informations about the authors of this collection of articles at the end of this book. The editors (Ed.) of this book are no authors. They have not modified or extended the original texts.

Pictures published in this book can be under different licences than the GNU Free Documentation License. You can get detailed informations about the authors and licences of pictures at the end of this book.

The content of this book was generated collaboratively by volunteers. Please be advised that nothing found here has necessarily been reviewed by people with the expertise required to provide you with complete, accurate or reliable information. Some information in this book maybe misleading or wrong. The Publisher does not guarantee the validity of the information found here. If you need specific advice (f.e. in fields of medical, legal, financial, or risk management questions) please contact a professional who is licensed or knowledgeable in that area.

Any brand names and product names mentioned in this book are subject to trademark, brand or patent protection and are trademarks or registered trademarks of their respective holders. The use of brand names, product names, common names, trade names, product descriptions etc. even without a particular marking in this works is in no way to be construed to mean that such names may be regarded as unrestricted in respect of trademark and brand protection legislation and could thus be used by anyone.

Cover image: www.ingimage.com
Concerning the licence of the cover image please contact ingimage.

Publisher:
Part Press is a trademark of
International Book Market Service Ltd., 17 Rue Meldrum, Beau Bassin, 1713-01 Mauritius
Email: info@bookmarketservice.com
Website: www.bookmarketservice.com

Published in 2013

Printed in: U.S.A., U.K., Germany. This book was not produced in Mauritius.

ISBN: 978-613-7-94558-2

Contents

Articles

References

Recessive

In genetics, a **recessive gene** is an allele that causes a phenotype (visible or detectable characteristic) that is only seen in a homozygous genotype (an organism that has two copies of the same allele) and never in a heterozygous genotype. Every person has two copies of every gene on autosomal chromosomes, one from mother and one from father. If a genetic trait is recessive, a person needs to inherit two copies of the gene for the trait to be expressed. Thus, both parents have to be carriers of a recessive trait in order for a child to express that trait. Note that "expression" in this sense does not refer to *genetic* expression (i.e., transcription and translation) of the gene. Instead, "expression" here refers to the observance of the gene within the phenotype. If both parents are carriers, there is a 25% chance with each child to show the recessive trait in the phenotype. Thus if the parents are closely related (in-breeding) the probability of both having inherited the same gene is increased and as a result the probability of the children showing the recessive trait is increased as well.

The term "recessive gene" is part of the laws of Mendelian inheritance created by Gregor Mendel. Examples of recessive genes in Mendel's famous pea plant experiments include those that determine the color and shape of seed pods, and plant height.

Allosomal recessive gene

Allosomal recessive is a mode of inheritance of genetic traits located on the allosomes (the sex determining chromosomes).

Examples include the gene for haemophilia which is carried on the X chromosome. Diseases carried on the Y chromosome cannot be recessive.

X chromosome diseases are recessive in females unless both of their X chromosomes have the gene. They are not recessive in males because males only have 1 X chromosome so there is not a non-diseased version of the gene to default to.

Autosomal recessive gene

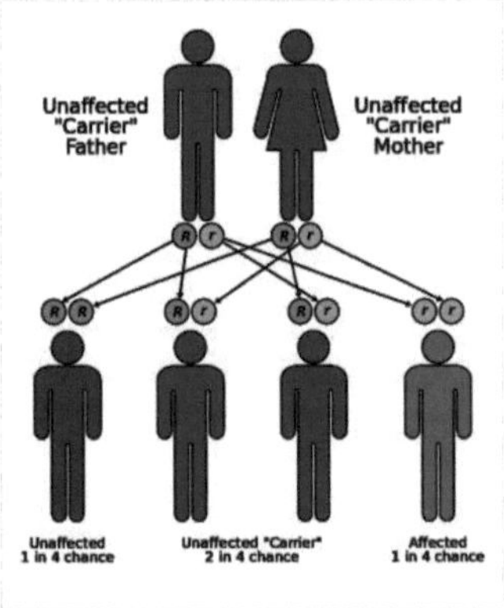

Autosomal recessive or **autorecessive** is a mode of inheritance of genetic traits located on the autosomes (the 22 non-sex determining chromosomes).

In opposition to autosomal dominant trait, a *recessive* trait only becomes phenotypically apparent when two copies of a gene (two alleles) are present. In other words, the subject is homozygous for the trait. Recessive genes will also show a horizontal inheritance on a pedigree chart. The frequency of the carrier state can be calculated by the Hardy-Weinberg formula: (p is the frequency of one allele, and $q = 1 - p$ is the frequency of the other allele. Thus $p*p$ is the frequency of the homozygous genotype for the first allele, $2pq$ is the frequency of the heterozygous genotype, and qq is the frequency of the other homozygous genotype.)

Recessive genetic disorders occur when both parents are carriers and each contributes an allele to the embryo. As both parents are heterozygous for the disorder, the chance of two disease alleles being inherited by one of their offspring is 25% (in autosomal dominant traits this is higher). 50% of the children (or 2/3 of the remaining ones) are carriers. When one of the parents is homozygous, the trait will only show in his/her offspring if the other parent is also a carrier. In that case, the chance of disease in the offspring is 50%.

Nomenclature

Technically, the term "recessive gene" is imprecise because it is not the gene that is recessive but the phenotype (or trait). It should also be noted that the concepts of recessiveness and dominance were developed before a molecular understanding of DNA and before molecular biology, thus mapping many newer concepts to "dominant" or "recessive" phenotypes is problematic. Many traits previously thought to be recessive have mild forms or biochemical abnormalities that arise from the presence of the one copy of the allele. This suggests that the dominant phenotype is dependent upon having two dominant genes and the presence of one dominant and one recessive gene creates some blending of both dominant and recessive traits.

	T	t
T	TT	Tt
t	Tt	tt

Recessive genes are usually represented by a lowercase letter in a Punnett square, as opposed to the uppercase letters of dominant genes (see example at right). Using the letter "T" as an example, only in "tt" (the homozygous recessive genotype, indicated by blue) would the recessive physical trait appear. The form "Tt" is called heterozygous (indicated by magenta with a red border), and, even though a recessive allele is present, the dominant gene is the one that appears (becomes the phenotype). The homozygous dominant genotype is "TT" (indicated by red)

Examples

Pea Plant

Gregor Mendel performed a multitude of experiments on pea plants (*Pisum sativum*) while researching traits, chosen because of the simple and low variety of characteristics, as well as the short period of germination. He experimented with color (green or yellow), size (short or tall), pea texture (smooth or wrinkled), and many others. By good fortune, the characteristics displayed by these plants clearly exhibited a dominant and recessive form. This is not true for many organisms. Few do inherit these traits.

For example, when testing the color of the pea plants, he chose two green plants, since green was more common than yellow. He mated them, and examined the offspring. He continued to mate only those that appeared green, and eventually, the yellow ones would stop being produced. He also mated the yellow ones together and determined that only yellow ones were produced.

Mendel determined that this was because yellow was a recessive trait which only appeared when green, the dominant trait, was not present. Also, he determined that the dominant trait would be displayed whether or not the recessive trait was there.

Autosomal recessive disease

Dominance/recessiveness refers to phenotype, not genotype. An example to prove the point is sickle cell anemia. The genotype of sickle cell is caused by a single base pair change in the beta-globin gene: normal=GAG (glu), sickle=GTG (val). There are several phenotypes associated with the sickle genotype: -

1. anemia (a recessive trait)
2. blood cell sickling (co-dominant)
3. altered beta-globin electrophoretic mobility (co-dominant)
4. resistance to malaria (dominant)

This example demonstrates that one can only refer to dominance/recessiveness with respect to individual phenotypes.

Other recessive disorders:

- Cystic fibrosis
- PKAN/NBIA
- Tay-Sachs disease
- Chronic granulomatous disease
- Thalassemia
- Bloom's Syndrome
- Alpha 1-antitrypsin deficiency
- Haemochromatosis types 1-3
- Wilson's disease
- Most types of Mucopolysaccharidosis
- Most Glycogen storage diseases
- Homocystinuria
- Congenital adrenal hyperplasia
- Dubin-Johnson syndrome
- Fanconi anemia
- Galactosemia
- Glucose-6-phosphate dehydrogenase deficiency
- Phenylketonuria
- Albinism
- Rotor syndrome
- Familial Mediterranean fever
- Pendred syndrome
- Certain forms of Spinal muscular atrophy
- Xeroderma pigmentosum
- Friedrich's ataxia

See also

- Dominant gene
- Incomplete dominance
- Dominance relationship
- X-linked
- mitochondrial

Spinal muscular atrophy

Spinal muscular atrophy

Classification and external resources

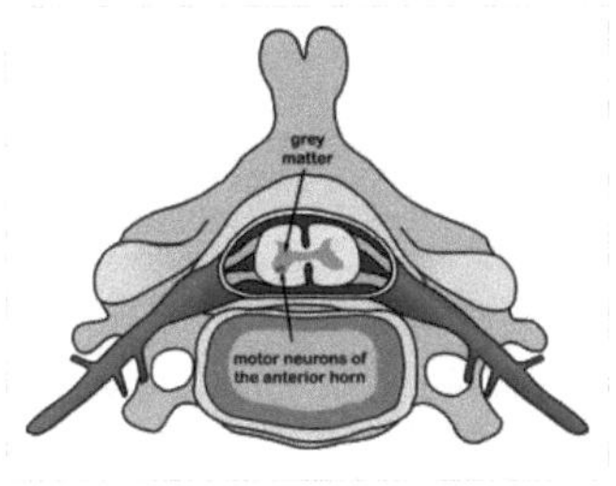

Location of neurons affected by spinal muscular atrophy in the spinal cord

ICD-10	G12.0 [1]-G12.1 [2]
ICD-9	335.0 [3]-335.1 [4]
OMIM	253300 [5] 253550 [6] 253400 [7] 271150 [8]
DiseasesDB	14093 [9] 32911 [10] 12315 [11] 34537 [12]
MedlinePlus	000996 [13]
eMedicine	Spinal Muscular Atrophy [14] Spinal Muscle Atrophy [15] Kugelberg–Welander SMA [16]
MeSH	[17]
GeneReviews	• Spinal Muscular Atrophy [18]

Spinal muscular atrophy (SMA) is an autosomal recessive disease caused by a genetic defect in the SMN1 gene that codes SMN, a protein widely expressed in all eukaryotic cells. SMN1 is apparently selectively necessary for survival of motor neurons, as diminished abundance of the protein results in death of neuronal cells in the anterior horn of spinal cord and subsequent system-wide muscle wasting (atrophy).

Spinal muscular atrophy manifests in various degrees of severity which all have in common general muscle wasting and mobility impairment. Other body systems may be affected as well, particularly in early-onset forms. SMA is the most common genetic cause of infant death.

The term *spinal muscular atrophy* is used as both a specific term for the genetic disorder caused by deficient SMN, and a general label for a larger number of rare disorders having in common a genetic cause and slow progression of weakness without sensory impairment caused by disease of motor neurons in the spinal cord and brainstem – see spinal muscular atrophies for a comparison chart.

Types

SMA manifests over a wide range of severity affecting infants through adults. The disease spectrum is variously divided into 3–5 types, in accordance either with the age of onset of symptoms or with the highest attained milestone of motor development.

The most commonly used classification is as follows:

Type	Eponym	Usual age of onset	Characteristics	OMIM
I: Infantile	Werdnig–Hoffmann disease	0–6 months	The severe form manifests in the first months of life, usually with a quick and unexpected onset ("floppy baby syndrome"). Rapid motor neuron death causes inefficiency of the major bodily organs - especially of the respiratory system - and pneumonia-induced respiratory failure is the most frequent cause of death. Babies diagnosed with SMA type I do not generally live past two years of age, with death occurring as early as within weeks in the most severe cases (sometimes termed *SMA type 0*). With proper respiratory support, those with milder SMA type I phenotypes, which account for around 10% of cases, are known to live into adolescence and adulthood.	253300 [5]
II: Intermediate	Dubowitz disease	6–18 months	The intermediate form affects children who are never able to stand and walk but who are able to maintain a sitting position at least some time in their life. The onset of weakness is usually noticed some time between 6 and 18 months. The progress is known to vary greatly, some patients gradually grow weaker over time while others through careful maintenance avoid any progression. Body muscles are weakened, and the respiratory system is a major concern. Life expectancy is somewhat reduced but most SMA II patients live well into adulthood.	253550 [6]
III: Juvenile	Kugelberg–Welander disease	>18 months	The juvenile form usually manifests after 18 months of age and describes patients who are able to walk without support at some time, although many later lose this ability. Respiratory involvement is less noticeable, and life expectancy is normal or near normal.	253400 [7]
IV: Adult-onset		Adulthood	The adult-onset form (sometimes classified as a late-onset SMA type III) usually manifests after the third decade of life with gradual weakening of muscles – mainly affects proximal muscles of the extremities – frequently rendering the patient wheelchair-bound. Other complications are rare, and life expectancy is unaffected.	271150 [8]

The most severe form of SMA type I is sometimes termed *SMA type 0* (or *severe infantile SMA*) and is diagnosed in babies that are born so weak that are able to survive only a few weeks even with intensive respiratory support. SMA type 0 should not be confused with SMARD1 which may have very similar symptoms and course but has a different genetic cause than SMA.

Development milestone attainment is commonly measured using a specially modified Hammersmith Functional Motor Scale.[19] [20] [21] [22]

The eponymous label *Werdnig-Hoffmann disease* (often misspelled with a single "n") refers to the earliest clinical descriptions of childhood SMA by Johann Hoffmann and Guido Werdnig. The eponymous term *Kugelberg-Welander disease* after Erik Klas Hendrik Kugelberg (1913-1983) and Lisa Welander (1909-2001), who distinguished SMA from muscular dystrophy. [23] Rarely used *Dubowitz disease* (not to be confused with Dubowitz syndrome) is named after Victor Dubowitz, an English neurologist who authored several studies on the intermediate SMA phenotype.

Causes

Spinal muscular atrophy is linked to a genetic mutation in the SMN1 gene.[24]

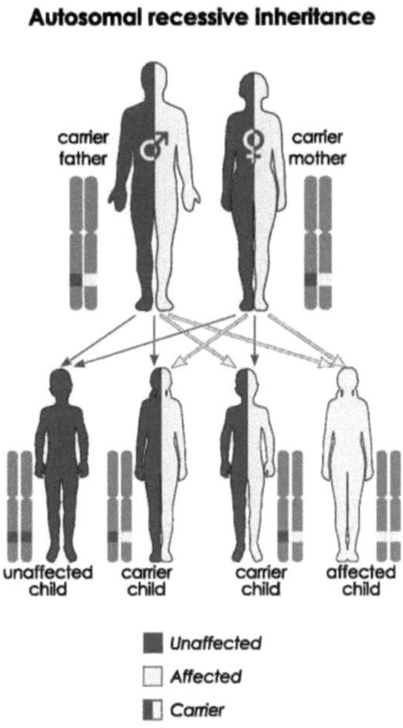

Spinal muscular atrophy has an autosomal recessive pattern of inheritance.

Human chromosome 5 contains two nearly identical genes at location 5q13: a telomeric copy **SMN1** and a centromeric copy **SMN2**. In healthy individuals, the SMN1 gene codes the survival of motor neuron protein (SMN) which, as its name says, plays a crucial role in survival of motor neurons. The SMN2 gene, on the other hand - due to a variation in a single nucleotide (840.C→T) - undergoes alternative splicing at the junction of intron 6 to exon 8, with only 10-20% of SMN2 transcripts coding a fully functional survival of motor neuron protein (SMN-fl) and 80-90% of transcripts resulting in a truncated protein compound (SMNΔ7) which is rapidly degraded in the cell.

In SMA-affected individuals, the SMN1 gene is mutated in such a way that it is unable to correctly code the SMN protein - due to either a deletion occurring at exon 7 or to other point mutations (frequently resulting in the functional conversion of the SMN1 sequence into SMN2). All patients, however, retain at least one copy of the SMN2 gene (with most having 2-4 of them) which still code small amounts of SMN protein - around 10-20% of the normal level - allowing neurons to survive. In the long run, however, reduced availability of the SMN protein results in gradual death of motor neuron cells in the anterior horn of spinal cord and the brain. Consequently, motor muscles undergo progressive atrophy.

Muscles of lower extremities are usually affected first, followed by muscles of upper extremities, spine and neck and, in more severe cases, pulmonary and mastication muscles. Proximal muscles are always affected earlier and in a greater degree than distal.

The severity of SMA symptoms is broadly related to how well the remaining SMN2 genes can make up for the loss of SMN1. This is partly related to the number of SMN2 gene copies present on the chromosome. Whilst healthy individuals carry two SMN2 gene copies, SMA patients can have anything between 1 and 4 (or more) of them, with the greater the number of SMN2 copies the milder the disease severity. Thus, most SMA type I babies have one or two SMN2 copies; SMA II and III patients usually have at least three SMN2 copies; and SMA IV patients normally have at least four of them. However, the correlation between symptom severity and SMN2 copy number is not absolute and there seem to exist other factors impacting on the disease phenotype.[25]

Spinal muscular atrophy is inherited in an autosomal recessive pattern, which means that the defective gene is located on an autosome, and two copies of the defective gene - one from each parent - are required to inherit the disorder: the parents do not need to be themselves affected. SMA seems to appear *de novo* (i.e., without any hereditary causes) in around 2-4% of cases.

Spinal muscular atrophy affects individuals of all races, unlike other well known autosomal recessive disorders like sickle cell disease and cystic fibrosis which have significant differences in occurrence rate between races. The overall incidence of SMA, of all types and across all ethnic groups, is in the range of 1 per 10,000 individuals; the gene frequency is thus around 1:100, therefore, approximately one in 50 persons are carriers.[26] [27] There are no known health consequences of being a carrier, and presently the only way one may know to consider the possibility is if a relative is affected.

Symptoms

The symptoms vary greatly depending on the SMA type involved, the stage of the disease and individual factors and commonly include:

- Areflexia, particularly in extremities
- Overall muscle weakness, poor muscle tone, limpness or a tendency to flop (the "floppy baby" syndrome)
- Difficulty achieving developmental milestones, difficulty sitting/standing/walking
- In infants: adopting of a frog-leg position when sitting (hips abducted and knees flexed)
- Loss of strength of the pulmonary muscles: weak cough, weak cry (infants), accumulation of secretions in the lungs or throat, respiratory distress
- Bell-shaped torso (caused by using only abdominal muscles for respiration)
- Clenched fists with sweaty hands
- Head often tilted to one side, even when lying down
- Fasciculations (twitching) of the tongue
- Difficulty sucking or swallowing, poor feeding
- Arthrogryposis (multiple congenital contractures)
- Weight lower than normal

Diagnosis

Prenatal screening is controversial, because of its cost on the one hand, and the severity of the disease on the other hand. Some researchers have concluded that population screening for SMA is not cost-effective, at a cost of $5 million per case averted in USA.[28] Others conclude that SMA meets the criteria for screening programs and relevant testing should be offered to all couples.[29]

Very severe SMA (type 0/I) can be sometimes evident before birth - reduction in fetal movement in the final months of pregnancy; else, it manifests within the first few weeks or months of life when abnormally low muscle tone is observed (the "floppy baby syndrome").

Further, for all SMA types,

- Patient will present hypotonia associated with absent reflexes
- Electromyogram will show fibrillation and muscle denervation[30]
- Serum creatine kinase may be normal or increased
- Genetic testing will show bi-allelic deletion of exon 7 of the SMN1 gene – this is conclusive of the disease.

Treatment

There is no known cure for spinal muscular atrophy.

Palliative care

Care is symptomatic. Main areas of concern are as follows:

- **Orthopaedics** — Weak spine muscles may lead to development of kyphosis, scoliosis and other orthopaedic problems. Spine fusion is sometimes performed in SMA I/II patients once they reach the age of 8-10 to relieve the pressure of a deformed spine on the lungs. SMA patients might also benefit greatly from various forms of physiotherapy and occupational therapy .
- **Respiratory care** — Respiratory system requires utmost attention in SMA as once weakened it never fully recovers. Weakened pulmonary muscles in SMA type I/II patients can make breathing more difficult and pose a

risk of hypoxiation, especially in sleep when muscles are more relaxed. Impaired cough reflex poses a constant risk of respiratory infection and pneumonia. Non-invasive ventilation (BiPAP) is frequently used and tracheostomy may be sometimes performed in more severe cases;[31] both methods of ventilation prolong survival in a comparable degree, although tracheostomy prevents speech development.[32]

- **Nutritional care** — Difficulties in jaw opening, chewing and swallowing food might pose SMA patients at risk of malnutrition. A feeding tube can be necessary in SMA type I and more severe type II patients.[33] [34] [35] Additionally, metabolic abnormalities resulting from SMA impair β-oxidation of fatty acids in muscles and can lead to organic acidemia and consequent muscle damage, especially when fasting.[36] [37] It is suggested that SMA patients, especially those with more severe forms of disease, reduce intake of fat and avoid prolonged fasting (i.e., eat more frequently than healthy people).[38]
- **Mobility** — Assistive technologies may help in managing movement and daily activity and greatly increase the quality of life.
- **Cardiology** — Although heart is not a matter of routine concern, a link between SMA and certain heart conditions has been suggested.[39] [40] [41] [42]
- **Mental health** — SMA children do not differ from the general population in their behaviour; their cognitive development can be slightly faster, and certain aspects of their intelligence are above the average.[43] [44] [45] Despite their disability, SMA-affected people report high degree of satisfaction from life.[46]

Palliative care in SMA has been standardised in the *Consensus Statement for Standard of Care in Spinal Muscular Atrophy* [47] which has been recommended for standard adoption worldwide.

Emerging therapies

Since the underlying genetic mechanism of SMA was described in 1990, several therapeutic approaches have been proposed and investigated. Since a vast number of *in vitro* and animal modelling studies suggest that restoration of SMN levels reverts SMA symptoms, the majority of emerging therapies focus on increasing the availability of SMN protein to motor neurons.

The main therapeutic pathways under research as of December 2011 include:[48] [49] [50] [51] [52] [52] [53] [53] [54]

- **Gene therapy** — aims at correcting the SMN1 gene function through inserting specially crafted nucleotide sequences with the help of a viral vector.[55] In the context of SMA, it is currently being researched using the scAAV9 viral vector at the Ohio State University and Nationwide Children's Hospital, USA, and the University of Sheffield, United Kingdom, as well as by Genzyme Corporation, USA, and Généthon, France. In one study this method has resulted in the greatest survival increase achieved to-date in a *SMNΔ7* mouse model (median survival of 400 days in treated mice as opposed to 15 days in untreated mice). Safety and pharmacokinetics of scAAV9 viral vector has been tested in non-human primates.[56]
- **Stem cell therapy** — aims at offering protection to affected neurons through injection of specially prepared human stem cells in the spinal cord which subsequently develop into neuronal cells able to code full-length SMN protein, and is developed commercially in the context of SMA by California Stem Cell, USA. Experimental stem cell therapy is also offered to SMA patients - based on limited research and with unclear outcome - in private clinics in Brazil, China, Russia, Ukraine and Lebanon.
- **SMN2 activation** — aims at increasing expression of the SMN2 gene and thus increasing the amount of full-length SMN available; compounds under investigation include:
    - Growth hormone
    - Histone deacetylase inhibitors:[57]
        - Aliphatic compounds:
            - Butyrates: sodium butyrate and sodium phenylbutyrate — promising *in vitro* and demonstrated effective in mouse models,[58] [59] [60] proved ineffective in symptomatic SMA patients (probably due to extremely short half-life),[61] still being trialled in pre-symptomatic type I/II infants[62]

    - Valproic acid — formerly used widely on experimental basis due to earlier research showing its effectiveness *in vitro*[63] and in mouse models,[64] in achievable concentrations demonstrated ineffective in SMA patients[65] [66] [67] and even shown to aggravate SMA symptoms[68]
  - Benzamides:
    - M344 — shown very effective in mouse models,[69] so far not trialled in SMA patients
  - Hydroxamic acids:
    - CBHA, SBHA — shown very promising *in vitro*
    - Entinostat (MS-275) — shown very promising *in vitro*
    - Panobinostat (LBH-589) — shown very effective in mouse models,[70] not trialled in SMA patients due to toxicity at required dosage
    - Trichostatin A — shown effective in mouse models,[71] [72] so far not trialled in SMA patients
    - Vorinostat (SAHA) — shown effective in mouse models,[73] so far not trialled in SMA patients
  - Hydroxycarbamide (hydroxyurea) — shown effective in mouse models[74] and subsequently commercially researched by Novo Nordisk, Denmark, but demonstrated no effect on SMA patients in subsequent clinical trials[75]
  - Natural polyphenol compounds: resveratrol, curcumin — moderate effectiveness on muscle strength supported by anecdotal evidence from patients and limited research *in vitro*[76] [77]
  - Prolactin — recently shown effective in mouse models,[78] so far not trialled in SMA patients
  - Salbutamol (albuterol) — demonstrated moderately effective *in vitro*[79] and in two clinical trials involving SMA II/III patients[80] [81]
- **SMN2 alternative splicing modulation** — targets the alternative splicing of the SMN2 gene so as to achieve a higher proportion of full-length SMN transcripts (sometimes called "gene conversion SMN2→SMN1"); compounds under investigation include:
  - Aclarubicin — shown effective in human cells from type I SMA patients,[82] not trialled any further due to toxicity at required dosage
  - Antisense oligonucleotides:[83] [84] [85]
    - *ISIS-SMNx* — a proprietary molecule under development by Isis Pharmaceuticals, USA, and as of July 2012, posed for a phase II clinical trial; has *Fast Track Designation* in the USA and *Orphan Medicinal Product Recommendation* in the European Union
    - *PTK-SMA1* — a proprietary small molecule splicing modulator of the tetracyclines group under development by Paratek Pharmaceutical, USA
  - Quinazolines:[86]
    - *RG3039* (formerly, *Quinazoline495*) — a proprietary quinazoline derivative under development by Repligen Corporation, USA, and as of July 2012, scheduled for phase II clinical trial; has an *Orphan Drug Designation* and *Fast Track Designation* in the USA and *Orphan Medicinal Product Recommendation* in the European Union
  - Sodium orthovanadate — shown to modulate alternative splicing in one study *in vitro*[87]
- **SMN stabilisation** — aims at stabilising the SMNΔ7 protein (the short-lived defective protein coded by the SMN2 gene) so that it is able to sustain neuronal cells;[88] investigated compounds include:
  - Aminoglycosides — shown to increase SMN protein availability[89] [90]
    - *TC-007* — a proprietary aminoglycoside antibiotic under commercial development by Tikvah Therapeutics, USA
  - Indoprofen[91]

- **Neuroprotection** — aims at prolonging survival of motor neurons even with low levels of SMN; investigated compounds include:
  - β-lactam antibiotics (e.g., ceftriaxone) — shown promising *in vitro*[92] [93]
  - Follistatin — shown promising *in vitro*[94]
  - Olesoxime — a proprietary compound developed by a French company Trophos, currently (2011-2013) under a phase II clinical trial in USA and Europe
  - Riluzole — a compound approved for treatment of ALS, currently being investigated for SMA at University of Angers, France
  - Thyrotropin-releasing hormone (TRH) — shown promising *in vitro* and in open-label uncontrolled clinical trials[95] [96] [97] yet did not prove effective in double-blind placebo-controlled trials[52]
- An unclear mechanism of action is found in the following compounds currently under research:
  - *PTC-X* — three proprietary compounds under joint development by PTC Therapeutics, USA, and Hoffmann-La Roche, Switzerland[98]
  - *RE-003* — a compound being developed by Retrophin.[99]

In vivo research is usually conducted using genetically engineered *Caenorhabditis elegans*,[100] [101] *Drosophila*,[100] [102] [103] zebrafish[104] and mouse[105] models; larger animal models are under development.[106] SMA patients can have a chance of participating in research by entering their details into international SMA patient registries [107]. A list of clinical trials targeting SMA can be found here [108].

It has to be noted, though, that SMA therapeutics seem to be most effective when given immediately after birth, then losing their efficacy with the patient's age. This might be related to the variation in time of the needs for SMN protein by neuronal cells. However, this also poses a major therapeutic problem as hardly ever is SMA diagnosed at birth.[109] [110]

Prognosis

Generally, patients tend to deteriorate over time, but prognosis varies with the SMA type and disease progress which shows a great degree of individual variability.

The majority of children diagnosed with SMA type 0/I do not reach the age of 10, recurrent respiratory problems being the primary cause of morbidity.[111] With proper care, milder SMA type I cases have lived into adulthood.[112]

In SMA type II, the course of the disease is stable or slowly progressing and life expectancy is somewhat reduced compared to the healthy population, although patients usually live to become parents and grandparents.

SMA type III has normal or nearly normal life expectancy if standards of care are followed. Adult-onset SMA usually means only mobility impairment and does not affect life expectancy.

External links

- Standards of Care in Spinal Muscular Atrophy [47]

See also

- SMA Treatment Acceleration Act
- Spinal muscular atrophies
- Motor neuron disease
- Survival of motor neuron
- Spinal muscular atrophy with respiratory distress type 1
- Spinal and bulbar muscular atrophy

References

[1] http://apps.who.int/classifications/icd10/browse/2010/en#/G12.0
[2] http://apps.who.int/classifications/icd10/browse/2010/en#/G12.1
[3] http://www.icd9data.com/getICD9Code.ashx?icd9=335.0
[4] http://www.icd9data.com/getICD9Code.ashx?icd9=335.1
[5] http://omim.org/entry/253300
[6] http://omim.org/entry/253550
[7] http://omim.org/entry/253400
[8] http://omim.org/entry/271150
[9] http://www.diseasesdatabase.com/ddb14093.htm
[10] http://www.diseasesdatabase.com/ddb32911.htm
[11] http://www.diseasesdatabase.com/ddb12315.htm
[12] http://www.diseasesdatabase.com/ddb34537.htm
[13] http://www.nlm.nih.gov/medlineplus/ency/article/000996.htm
[14] http://emedicine.medscape.com/article/1181436-overview
[15] http://emedicine.medscape.com/article/1264401-overview
[16] http://emedicine.medscape.com/article/306812-overview
[17] http://www.nlm.nih.gov/cgi/mesh//MB_cgi?
[18] http://www.ncbi.nlm.nih.gov/books/NBK1352/
[19] Error: Bad DOI specified!
[20] Error: Bad DOI specified!
[21] Error: Bad DOI specified!
[22] Error: Bad DOI specified!
[23] Error: Bad DOI specified!
[24] Error: Bad DOI specified!
[25] Jędrzejowska, M.; Milewski, M.; Zimowski, J.; Borkowska, J.; Kostera-Pruszczyk, A.; Sielska, D.; Jurek, M.; Hausmanowa-Petrusewicz, I. (2009). "Phenotype modifiers of spinal muscular atrophy: The number of SMN2 gene copies, deletion in the NAIP gene and probably gender influence the course of the disease". *Acta Biochimica Polonica* **56** (1): 103–108. PMID 19287802.
[26] Error: Bad DOI specified!
[27] Error: Bad DOI specified!
[28] Error: Bad DOI specified!
[29] Error: Bad DOI specified!
[30] Error: Bad DOI specified!
[31] Error: Bad DOI specified!
[32] Error: Bad DOI specified!
[33] Error: Bad DOI specified!
[34] Error: Bad DOI specified!
[35] Error: Bad DOI specified!
[36] Tein, I.; Sloane, A. E.; Donner, E. J.; Lehotay, D. C.; Millington, D. S.; Kelley, R. I. (1995). "Fatty acid oxidation abnormalities in childhood-onset spinal muscular atrophy: Primary or secondary defect(s)?". *Pediatric neurology* **12** (1): 21–30. doi:10.1016/0887-8994(94)00100-G. PMID 7748356.
[37] Crawford, T. O.; Sladky, J. T.; Hurko, O.; Besner-Johnston, A.; Kelley, R. I. (1999). "Abnormal fatty acid metabolism in childhood spinal muscular atrophy". *Annals of neurology* **45** (3): 337–343. doi:10.1002/1531-8249(199903)45:3<337::AID-ANA9>3.0.CO;2-U. PMID 10072048.
[38] Leighton, S. (2003). "Nutrition issues associated with spinal muscular atrophy". *Nutrition & Dietetics* **60** (2): 92–96.
[39] Error: Bad DOI specified!
[40] Error: Bad DOI specified!
[41] Error: Bad DOI specified!
[42] Error: Bad DOI specified!
[43] Error: Bad DOI specified!
[44] Error: Bad DOI specified!
[45] Error: Bad DOI specified!
[46] Error: Bad DOI specified!
[47] http://dx.doi.org/10.1177/0883073807305788
[48] Error: Bad DOI specified!
[49] Error: Bad DOI specified!
[50] Error: Bad DOI specified!
[51] Error: Bad DOI specified!

[52] Error: Bad DOI specified!
[53] Error: Bad DOI specified!
[54] Error: Bad DOI specified!
[55] Error: Bad DOI specified!
[56] Error: Bad DOI specified!
[57] Error: Bad DOI specified!
[58] Error: Bad DOI specified!
[59] Error: Bad DOI specified!
[60] Error: Bad DOI specified!
[61] Error: Bad DOI specified!
[62] "Study to Evaluate Sodium Phenylbutyrate in Pre-symptomatic Infants With Spinal Muscular Atrophy (STOPSMA)" (http://clinicaltrials.gov/ct2/show/NCT00528268). . Retrieved 28 December 2011.
[63] Error: Bad DOI specified!
[64] Error: Bad DOI specified!
[65] Error: Bad DOI specified!
[66] Error: Bad DOI specified!
[67] Error: Bad DOI specified!
[68] Error: Bad DOI specified!
[69] Error: Bad DOI specified!
[70] Error: Bad DOI specified!
[71] Error: Bad DOI specified!
[72] Error: Bad DOI specified!
[73] Error: Bad DOI specified!
[74] Error: Bad DOI specified!
[75] Error: Bad DOI specified!
[76] Error: Bad DOI specified!
[77] Error: Bad DOI specified!
[78] Error: Bad DOI specified!
[79] Error: Bad DOI specified!
[80] Error: Bad DOI specified!
[81] Error: Bad DOI specified!
[82] Error: Bad DOI specified!
[83] Error: Bad DOI specified!
[84] Error: Bad DOI specified!
[85] Error: Bad DOI specified!
[86] Error: Bad DOI specified!
[87] Error: Bad DOI specified!
[88] Error: Bad DOI specified!
[89] Error: Bad DOI specified!
[90] Error: Bad DOI specified!
[91] Error: Bad DOI specified!
[92] Error: Bad DOI specified!
[93] Error: Bad DOI specified!
[94] Error: Bad DOI specified!
[95] Error: Bad DOI specified!
[96] Tzeng, A. C.; Cheng, J.; Fryczynski, H.; Niranjan, V.; Stitik, T.; Sial, A.; Takeuchi, Y.; Foye, P. et al. (2000). "A study of thyrotropin-releasing hormone for the treatment of spinal muscular atrophy: A preliminary report". *American journal of physical medicine & rehabilitation / Association of Academic Physiatrists* **79** (5): 435–440. PMID 10994885.
[97] Error: Bad DOI specified!
[98] "Roche signs agreement with PTC Therapeutics to advance treatment for Spinal Muscular Atrophy (SMA)" (http://ptct.client.shareholder.com/ReleaseDetail.cfm?ReleaseID=627602). . Retrieved 28 December 2011.
[99] "Rethropin: drug pipeline" (http://www.retrophin.com/pipeline.php). . Retrieved 08 May 2012.
[100] Error: Bad DOI specified!
[101] Error: Bad DOI specified!
[102] Error: Bad DOI specified!
[103] Error: Bad DOI specified!
[104] Error: Bad DOI specified!
[105] Error: Bad DOI specified!

[106] "The GSF and FightSMA Announce 100K Research Award for the Development of a Large Animal Model of Spinal Muscular Atrophy" (http://www.fightsma.org/blog/uncategorized/the-gsf-and-fightsma-announce-100k-research-award). . Retrieved 18 December 2011.
[107] http://www.treat-nmd.eu/resources/patient-registries/national-registries
[108] http://clinicaltrials.gov/ct2/results?term=spinal+muscular+atrophy
[109] Error: Bad DOI specified!
[110] Error: Bad DOI specified!
[111] Error: Bad DOI specified!
[112] Error: Bad DOI specified!

Survival motor neuron spinal muscular atrophy

Spinal muscular atrophy	
Classification and external resources	

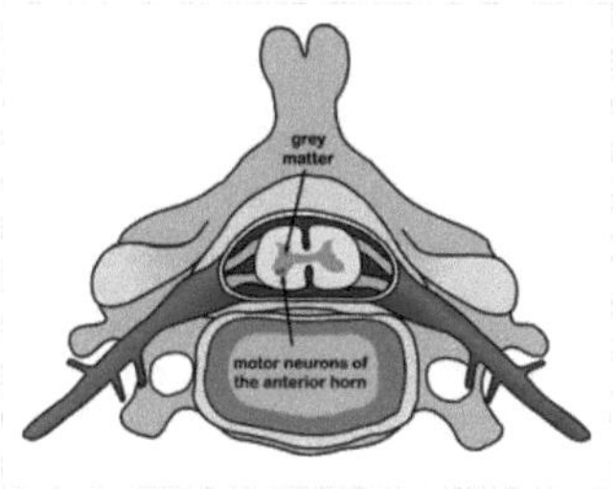

Location of neurons affected by spinal muscular atrophy in the spinal cord

ICD-10	G12.0 [1]-G12.1 [2]
ICD-9	335.0 [3]-335.1 [4]
OMIM	253300 [5] 253550 [6] 253400 [7] 271150 [8]
DiseasesDB	14093 [9] 32911 [10] 12315 [11] 34537 [12]
MedlinePlus	000996 [13]
eMedicine	Spinal Muscular Atrophy [14] Spinal Muscle Atrophy [15] Kugelberg–Welander SMA [16]
MeSH	[17]
GeneReviews	• Spinal Muscular Atrophy [18]

Spinal muscular atrophy (SMA) is an autosomal recessive disease caused by a genetic defect in the SMN1 gene that codes SMN, a protein widely expressed in all eukaryotic cells. SMN1 is apparently selectively necessary for survival of motor neurons, as diminished abundance of the protein results in death of neuronal cells in the anterior horn of spinal cord and subsequent system-wide muscle wasting (atrophy).

Spinal muscular atrophy manifests in various degrees of severity which all have in common general muscle wasting and mobility impairment. Other body systems may be affected as well, particularly in early-onset forms. SMA is the most common genetic cause of infant death.

The term *spinal muscular atrophy* is used as both a specific term for the genetic disorder caused by deficient SMN, and a general label for a larger number of rare disorders having in common a genetic cause and slow progression of weakness without sensory impairment caused by disease of motor neurons in the spinal cord and brainstem – see spinal muscular atrophies for a comparison chart.

Types

SMA manifests over a wide range of severity affecting infants through adults. The disease spectrum is variously divided into 3–5 types, in accordance either with the age of onset of symptoms or with the highest attained milestone of motor development.

The most commonly used classification is as follows:

Type	Eponym	Usual age of onset	Characteristics	OMIM
I: Infantile	Werdnig–Hoffmann disease	0–6 months	The severe form manifests in the first months of life, usually with a quick and unexpected onset ("floppy baby syndrome"). Rapid motor neuron death causes inefficiency of the major bodily organs - especially of the respiratory system - and pneumonia-induced respiratory failure is the most frequent cause of death. Babies diagnosed with SMA type I do not generally live past two years of age, with death occurring as early as within weeks in the most severe cases (sometimes termed *SMA type 0*). With proper respiratory support, those with milder SMA type I phenotypes, which account for around 10% of cases, are known to live into adolescence and adulthood.	253300 [5]
II: Intermediate	Dubowitz disease	6–18 months	The intermediate form affects children who are never able to stand and walk but who are able to maintain a sitting position at least some time in their life. The onset of weakness is usually noticed some time between 6 and 18 months. The progress is known to vary greatly, some patients gradually grow weaker over time while others through careful maintenance avoid any progression. Body muscles are weakened, and the respiratory system is a major concern. Life expectancy is somewhat reduced but most SMA II patients live well into adulthood.	253550 [6]
III: Juvenile	Kugelberg–Welander disease	>18 months	The juvenile form usually manifests after 18 months of age and describes patients who are able to walk without support at some time, although many later lose this ability. Respiratory involvement is less noticeable, and life expectancy is normal or near normal.	253400 [7]
IV: Adult-onset		Adulthood	The adult-onset form (sometimes classified as a late-onset SMA type III) usually manifests after the third decade of life with gradual weakening of muscles – mainly affects proximal muscles of the extremities – frequently rendering the patient wheelchair-bound. Other complications are rare, and life expectancy is unaffected.	271150 [8]

The most severe form of SMA type I is sometimes termed *SMA type 0* (or *severe infantile SMA*) and is diagnosed in babies that are born so weak that are able to survive only a few weeks even with intensive respiratory support. SMA type 0 should not be confused with SMARD1 which may have very similar symptoms and course but has a different genetic cause than SMA.

Development milestone attainment is commonly measured using a specially modified Hammersmith Functional Motor Scale.[1] [2] [3] [4]

The eponymous label *Werdnig-Hoffmann disease* (often misspelled with a single "n") refers to the earliest clinical descriptions of childhood SMA by Johann Hoffmann and Guido Werdnig. The eponymous term *Kugelberg-Welander disease* after Erik Klas Hendrik Kugelberg (1913-1983) and Lisa Welander (1909-2001), who distinguished SMA from muscular dystrophy. [5] Rarely used *Dubowitz disease* (not to be confused with Dubowitz syndrome) is named after Victor Dubowitz, an English neurologist who authored several studies on the intermediate SMA phenotype.

Causes

Spinal muscular atrophy is linked to a genetic mutation in the SMN1 gene.[6]

Human chromosome 5 contains two nearly identical genes at location 5q13: a telomeric copy **SMN1** and a centromeric copy **SMN2**. In healthy individuals, the SMN1 gene codes the survival of motor neuron protein (SMN) which, as its name says, plays a crucial role in survival of motor neurons. The SMN2 gene, on the other hand - due to a variation in a single nucleotide (840.C→T) - undergoes alternative splicing at the junction of intron 6 to exon 8, with only 10-20% of SMN2 transcripts coding a fully functional survival of motor neuron protein (SMN-fl) and 80-90% of transcripts resulting in a truncated protein compound (SMNΔ7) which is rapidly degraded in the cell.

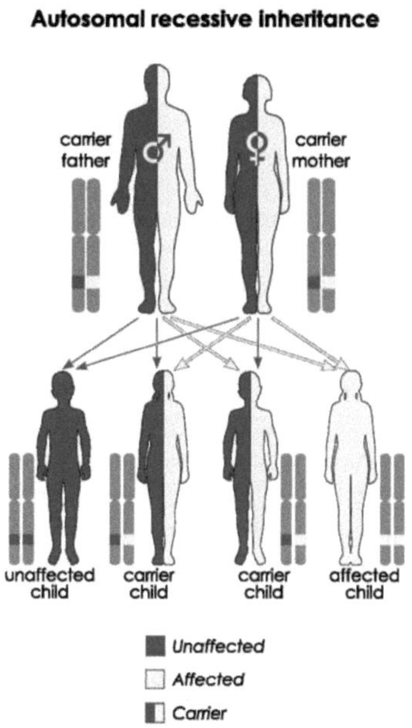

Spinal muscular atrophy has an autosomal recessive pattern of inheritance.

In SMA-affected individuals, the SMN1 gene is mutated in such a way that it is unable to correctly code the SMN protein - due to either a deletion occurring at exon 7 or to other point mutations (frequently resulting in the functional conversion of the SMN1 sequence into SMN2). All patients, however, retain at least one copy of the SMN2 gene (with most having 2-4 of them) which still code small amounts of SMN protein - around 10-20% of the normal level - allowing neurons to survive. In the long run, however, reduced availability of the SMN protein results in gradual death of motor neuron cells in the anterior horn of spinal cord and the brain. Consequently, motor muscles undergo progressive atrophy.

Muscles of lower extremities are usually affected first, followed by muscles of upper extremities, spine and neck and, in more severe cases, pulmonary and mastication muscles. Proximal muscles are always affected earlier and in a greater degree than distal.

The severity of SMA symptoms is broadly related to how well the remaining SMN2 genes can make up for the loss of SMN1. This is partly related to the number of SMN2 gene copies present on the chromosome. Whilst healthy individuals carry two SMN2 gene copies, SMA patients can have anything between 1 and 4 (or more) of them, with the greater the number of SMN2 copies the milder the disease severity. Thus, most SMA type I babies have one or two SMN2 copies; SMA II and III patients usually have at least three SMN2 copies; and SMA IV patients normally have at least four of them. However, the correlation between symptom severity and SMN2 copy number is not absolute and there seem to exist other factors impacting on the disease phenotype.[7]

Spinal muscular atrophy is inherited in an autosomal recessive pattern, which means that the defective gene is located on an autosome, and two copies of the defective gene - one from each parent - are required to inherit the disorder: the parents do not need to be themselves affected. SMA seems to appear *de novo* (i.e., without any hereditary causes) in around 2-4% of cases.

Spinal muscular atrophy affects individuals of all races, unlike other well known autosomal recessive disorders like sickle cell disease and cystic fibrosis which have significant differences in occurrence rate between races. The overall incidence of SMA, of all types and across all ethnic groups, is in the range of 1 per 10,000 individuals; the gene frequency is thus around 1:100, therefore, approximately one in 50 persons are carriers.[8] [9] There are no known health consequences of being a carrier, and presently the only way one may know to consider the possibility is if a relative is affected.

Symptoms

The symptoms vary greatly depending on the SMA type involved, the stage of the disease and individual factors and commonly include:

- Areflexia, particularly in extremities
- Overall muscle weakness, poor muscle tone, limpness or a tendency to flop (the "floppy baby" syndrome)
- Difficulty achieving developmental milestones, difficulty sitting/standing/walking
- In infants: adopting of a frog-leg position when sitting (hips abducted and knees flexed)
- Loss of strength of the pulmonary muscles: weak cough, weak cry (infants), accumulation of secretions in the lungs or throat, respiratory distress
- Bell-shaped torso (caused by using only abdominal muscles for respiration)
- Clenched fists with sweaty hands
- Head often tilted to one side, even when lying down
- Fasciculations (twitching) of the tongue
- Difficulty sucking or swallowing, poor feeding
- Arthrogryposis (multiple congenital contractures)
- Weight lower than normal

Diagnosis

Prenatal screening is controversial, because of its cost on the one hand, and the severity of the disease on the other hand. Some researchers have concluded that population screening for SMA is not cost-effective, at a cost of $5 million per case averted in USA.[10] Others conclude that SMA meets the criteria for screening programs and relevant testing should be offered to all couples.[11]

Very severe SMA (type 0/I) can be sometimes evident before birth - reduction in fetal movement in the final months of pregnancy; else, it manifests within the first few weeks or months of life when abnormally low muscle tone is observed (the "floppy baby syndrome").

Further, for all SMA types,

- Patient will present hypotonia associated with absent reflexes
- Electromyogram will show fibrillation and muscle denervation[12]
- Serum creatine kinase may be normal or increased
- Genetic testing will show bi-allelic deletion of exon 7 of the SMN1 gene – this is conclusive of the disease.

Treatment

There is no known cure for spinal muscular atrophy.

Palliative care

Care is symptomatic. Main areas of concern are as follows:

- **Orthopaedics** — Weak spine muscles may lead to development of kyphosis, scoliosis and other orthopaedic problems. Spine fusion is sometimes performed in SMA I/II patients once they reach the age of 8-10 to relieve the pressure of a deformed spine on the lungs. SMA patients might also benefit greatly from various forms of physiotherapy and occupational therapy .
- **Respiratory care** — Respiratory system requires utmost attention in SMA as once weakened it never fully recovers. Weakened pulmonary muscles in SMA type I/II patients can make breathing more difficult and pose a

risk of hypoxiation, especially in sleep when muscles are more relaxed. Impaired cough reflex poses a constant risk of respiratory infection and pneumonia. Non-invasive ventilation (BiPAP) is frequently used and tracheostomy may be sometimes performed in more severe cases;[13] both methods of ventilation prolong survival in a comparable degree, although tracheostomy prevents speech development.[14]

- **Nutritional care** — Difficulties in jaw opening, chewing and swallowing food might pose SMA patients at risk of malnutrition. A feeding tube can be necessary in SMA type I and more severe type II patients.[15] [16] [17] Additionally, metabolic abnormalities resulting from SMA impair β-oxidation of fatty acids in muscles and can lead to organic acidemia and consequent muscle damage, especially when fasting.[18] [19] It is suggested that SMA patients, especially those with more severe forms of disease, reduce intake of fat and avoid prolonged fasting (i.e., eat more frequently than healthy people).[20]
- **Mobility** — Assistive technologies may help in managing movement and daily activity and greatly increase the quality of life.
- **Cardiology** — Although heart is not a matter of routine concern, a link between SMA and certain heart conditions has been suggested.[21] [22] [23] [24]
- **Mental health** — SMA children do not differ from the general population in their behaviour; their cognitive development can be slightly faster, and certain aspects of their intelligence are above the average.[25] [26] [27] Despite their disability, SMA-affected people report high degree of satisfaction from life.[28]

Palliative care in SMA has been standardised in the *Consensus Statement for Standard of Care in Spinal Muscular Atrophy* [47] which has been recommended for standard adoption worldwide.

Emerging therapies

Since the underlying genetic mechanism of SMA was described in 1990, several therapeutic approaches have been proposed and investigated. Since a vast number of *in vitro* and animal modelling studies suggest that restoration of SMN levels reverts SMA symptoms, the majority of emerging therapies focus on increasing the availability of SMN protein to motor neurons.

The main therapeutic pathways under research as of December 2011 include:[29] [30] [31] [32] [33] [33] [34] [34] [35]

- **Gene therapy** — aims at correcting the SMN1 gene function through inserting specially crafted nucleotide sequences with the help of a viral vector.[36] In the context of SMA, it is currently being researched using the scAAV9 viral vector at the Ohio State University and Nationwide Children's Hospital, USA, and the University of Sheffield, United Kingdom, as well as by Genzyme Corporation, USA, and Généthon, France. In one study this method has resulted in the greatest survival increase achieved to-date in a *SMNΔ7* mouse model (median survival of 400 days in treated mice as opposed to 15 days in untreated mice). Safety and pharmacokinetics of scAAV9 viral vector has been tested in non-human primates.[37]
- **Stem cell therapy** — aims at offering protection to affected neurons through injection of specially prepared human stem cells in the spinal cord which subsequently develop into neuronal cells able to code full-length SMN protein, and is developed commercially in the context of SMA by California Stem Cell, USA. Experimental stem cell therapy is also offered to SMA patients - based on limited research and with unclear outcome - in private clinics in Brazil, China, Russia, Ukraine and Lebanon.
- **SMN2 activation** — aims at increasing expression of the SMN2 gene and thus increasing the amount of full-length SMN available; compounds under investigation include:
    - Growth hormone
    - Histone deacetylase inhibitors:[38]
        - Aliphatic compounds:
            - Butyrates: sodium butyrate and sodium phenylbutyrate — promising *in vitro* and demonstrated effective in mouse models,[39] [40] [41] proved ineffective in symptomatic SMA patients (probably due to extremely short half-life),[42] still being trialled in pre-symptomatic type I/II infants[43]

    - Valproic acid — formerly used widely on experimental basis due to earlier research showing its effectiveness *in vitro*[44] and in mouse models,[45] in achievable concentrations demonstrated ineffective in SMA patients[46] [47] [48] and even shown to aggravate SMA symptoms[49]
  - Benzamides:
    - M344 — shown very effective in mouse models,[50] so far not trialled in SMA patients
  - Hydroxamic acids:
    - CBHA, SBHA — shown very promising *in vitro*
    - Entinostat (MS-275) — shown very promising *in vitro*
    - Panobinostat (LBH-589) — shown very effective in mouse models,[51] not trialled in SMA patients due to toxicity at required dosage
    - Trichostatin A — shown effective in mouse models,[52] [53] so far not trialled in SMA patients
    - Vorinostat (SAHA) — shown effective in mouse models,[54] so far not trialled in SMA patients
  - Hydroxycarbamide (hydroxyurea) — shown effective in mouse models[55] and subsequently commercially researched by Novo Nordisk, Denmark, but demonstrated no effect on SMA patients in subsequent clinical trials[56]
  - Natural polyphenol compounds: resveratrol, curcumin — moderate effectiveness on muscle strength supported by anecdotal evidence from patients and limited research *in vitro*[57] [58]
  - Prolactin — recently shown effective in mouse models,[59] so far not trialled in SMA patients
  - Salbutamol (albuterol) — demonstrated moderately effective *in vitro*[60] and in two clinical trials involving SMA II/III patients[61] [62]
- **SMN2 alternative splicing modulation** — targets the alternative splicing of the SMN2 gene so as to achieve a higher proportion of full-length SMN transcripts (sometimes called "gene conversion SMN2→SMN1"); compounds under investigation include:
  - Aclarubicin — shown effective in human cells from type I SMA patients,[63] not trialled any further due to toxicity at required dosage
  - Antisense oligonucleotides:[64] [65] [66]
    - *ISIS-SMNx* — a proprietary molecule under development by Isis Pharmaceuticals, USA, and as of July 2012, posed for a phase II clinical trial; has *Fast Track Designation* in the USA and *Orphan Medicinal Product Recommendation* in the European Union
    - *PTK-SMA1* — a proprietary small molecule splicing modulator of the tetracyclines group under development by Paratek Pharmaceutical, USA
  - Quinazolines:[67]
    - *RG3039* (formerly, *Quinazoline495*) — a proprietary quinazoline derivative under development by Repligen Corporation, USA, and as of July 2012, scheduled for phase II clinical trial; has an *Orphan Drug Designation* and *Fast Track Designation* in the USA and *Orphan Medicinal Product Recommendation* in the European Union
  - Sodium orthovanadate — shown to modulate alternative splicing in one study *in vitro*[68]
- **SMN stabilisation** — aims at stabilising the SMNΔ7 protein (the short-lived defective protein coded by the SMN2 gene) so that it is able to sustain neuronal cells;[69] investigated compounds include:
  - Aminoglycosides — shown to increase SMN protein availability[70] [71]
    - *TC-007* — a proprietary aminoglycoside antibiotic under commercial development by Tikvah Therapeutics, USA
  - Indoprofen[72]

- **Neuroprotection** — aims at prolonging survival of motor neurons even with low levels of SMN; investigated compounds include:
  - β-lactam antibiotics (e.g., ceftriaxone) — shown promising *in vitro*[73] [74]
  - Follistatin — shown promising *in vitro*[75]
  - Olesoxime — a proprietary compound developed by a French company Trophos, currently (2011-2013) under a phase II clinical trial in USA and Europe
  - Riluzole — a compound approved for treatment of ALS, currently being investigated for SMA at University of Angers, France
  - Thyrotropin-releasing hormone (TRH) — shown promising *in vitro* and in open-label uncontrolled clinical trials[76] [77] [78] yet did not prove effective in double-blind placebo-controlled trials[33]
- An unclear mechanism of action is found in the following compounds currently under research:
  - *PTC-X* — three proprietary compounds under joint development by PTC Therapeutics, USA, and Hoffmann-La Roche, Switzerland[79]
  - *RE-003* — a compound being developed by Retrophin.[80]

In vivo research is usually conducted using genetically engineered *Caenorhabditis elegans*,[81] [82] *Drosophila*,[81] [83] [84] zebrafish[85] and mouse[86] models; larger animal models are under development.[87] SMA patients can have a chance of participating in research by entering their details into international SMA patient registries [107]. A list of clinical trials targeting SMA can be found here [108].

It has to be noted, though, that SMA therapeutics seem to be most effective when given immediately after birth, then losing their efficacy with the patient's age. This might be related to the variation in time of the needs for SMN protein by neuronal cells. However, this also poses a major therapeutic problem as hardly ever is SMA diagnosed at birth.[88] [89]

Prognosis

Generally, patients tend to deteriorate over time, but prognosis varies with the SMA type and disease progress which shows a great degree of individual variability.

The majority of children diagnosed with SMA type 0/I do not reach the age of 10, recurrent respiratory problems being the primary cause of morbidity.[90] With proper care, milder SMA type I cases have lived into adulthood.[91]

In SMA type II, the course of the disease is stable or slowly progressing and life expectancy is somewhat reduced compared to the healthy population, although patients usually live to become parents and grandparents.

SMA type III has normal or nearly normal life expectancy if standards of care are followed. Adult-onset SMA usually means only mobility impairment and does not affect life expectancy.

External links

- Standards of Care in Spinal Muscular Atrophy [47]

See also

- SMA Treatment Acceleration Act
- Spinal muscular atrophies
- Motor neuron disease
- Survival of motor neuron
- Spinal muscular atrophy with respiratory distress type 1
- Spinal and bulbar muscular atrophy

References

[1] Error: Bad DOI specified!
[2] Error: Bad DOI specified!
[3] Error: Bad DOI specified!
[4] Error: Bad DOI specified!
[5] Error: Bad DOI specified!
[6] Error: Bad DOI specified!
[7] Jędrzejowska, M.; Milewski, M.; Zimowski, J.; Borkowska, J.; Kostera-Pruszczyk, A.; Sielska, D.; Jurek, M.; Hausmanowa-Petrusewicz, I. (2009). "Phenotype modifiers of spinal muscular atrophy: The number of SMN2 gene copies, deletion in the NAIP gene and probably gender influence the course of the disease". *Acta Biochimica Polonica* **56** (1): 103–108. PMID 19287802.
[8] Error: Bad DOI specified!
[9] Error: Bad DOI specified!
[10] Error: Bad DOI specified!
[11] Error: Bad DOI specified!
[12] Error: Bad DOI specified!
[13] Error: Bad DOI specified!
[14] Error: Bad DOI specified!
[15] Error: Bad DOI specified!
[16] Error: Bad DOI specified!
[17] Error: Bad DOI specified!
[18] Tein, I.; Sloane, A. E.; Donner, E. J.; Lehotay, D. C.; Millington, D. S.; Kelley, R. I. (1995). "Fatty acid oxidation abnormalities in childhood-onset spinal muscular atrophy: Primary or secondary defect(s)?". *Pediatric neurology* **12** (1): 21–30. doi:10.1016/0887-8994(94)00100-G. PMID 7748356.
[19] Crawford, T. O.; Sladky, J. T.; Hurko, O.; Besner-Johnston, A.; Kelley, R. I. (1999). "Abnormal fatty acid metabolism in childhood spinal muscular atrophy". *Annals of neurology* **45** (3): 337–343. doi:10.1002/1531-8249(199903)45:3<337::AID-ANA9>3.0.CO;2-U. PMID 10072048.
[20] Leighton, S. (2003). "Nutrition issues associated with spinal muscular atrophy". *Nutrition & Dietetics* **60** (2): 92–96.
[21] Error: Bad DOI specified!
[22] Error: Bad DOI specified!
[23] Error: Bad DOI specified!
[24] Error: Bad DOI specified!
[25] Error: Bad DOI specified!
[26] Error: Bad DOI specified!
[27] Error: Bad DOI specified!
[28] Error: Bad DOI specified!
[29] Error: Bad DOI specified!
[30] Error: Bad DOI specified!
[31] Error: Bad DOI specified!
[32] Error: Bad DOI specified!
[33] Error: Bad DOI specified!
[34] Error: Bad DOI specified!
[35] Error: Bad DOI specified!
[36] Error: Bad DOI specified!
[37] Error: Bad DOI specified!
[38] Error: Bad DOI specified!
[39] Error: Bad DOI specified!
[40] Error: Bad DOI specified!
[41] Error: Bad DOI specified!
[42] Error: Bad DOI specified!
[43] "Study to Evaluate Sodium Phenylbutyrate in Pre-symptomatic Infants With Spinal Muscular Atrophy (STOPSMA)" (http://clinicaltrials.gov/ct2/show/NCT00528268). . Retrieved 28 December 2011.
[44] Error: Bad DOI specified!
[45] Error: Bad DOI specified!
[46] Error: Bad DOI specified!
[47] Error: Bad DOI specified!
[48] Error: Bad DOI specified!
[49] Error: Bad DOI specified!
[50] Error: Bad DOI specified!

[51] Error: Bad DOI specified!
[52] Error: Bad DOI specified!
[53] Error: Bad DOI specified!
[54] Error: Bad DOI specified!
[55] Error: Bad DOI specified!
[56] Error: Bad DOI specified!
[57] Error: Bad DOI specified!
[58] Error: Bad DOI specified!
[59] Error: Bad DOI specified!
[60] Error: Bad DOI specified!
[61] Error: Bad DOI specified!
[62] Error: Bad DOI specified!
[63] Error: Bad DOI specified!
[64] Error: Bad DOI specified!
[65] Error: Bad DOI specified!
[66] Error: Bad DOI specified!
[67] Error: Bad DOI specified!
[68] Error: Bad DOI specified!
[69] Error: Bad DOI specified!
[70] Error: Bad DOI specified!
[71] Error: Bad DOI specified!
[72] Error: Bad DOI specified!
[73] Error: Bad DOI specified!
[74] Error: Bad DOI specified!
[75] Error: Bad DOI specified!
[76] Error: Bad DOI specified!
[77] Tzeng, A. C.; Cheng, J.; Fryczynski, H.; Niranjan, V.; Stitik, T.; Sial, A.; Takeuchi, Y.; Foye, P. et al. (2000). "A study of thyrotropin-releasing hormone for the treatment of spinal muscular atrophy: A preliminary report". *American journal of physical medicine & rehabilitation / Association of Academic Physiatrists* **79** (5): 435–440. PMID 10994885.
[78] Error: Bad DOI specified!
[79] "Roche signs agreement with PTC Therapeutics to advance treatment for Spinal Muscular Atrophy (SMA)" (http://ptct.client.shareholder.com/ReleaseDetail.cfm?ReleaseID=627602). . Retrieved 28 December 2011.
[80] "Rethropin: drug pipeline" (http://www.retrophin.com/pipeline.php). . Retrieved 08 May 2012.
[81] Error: Bad DOI specified!
[82] Error: Bad DOI specified!
[83] Error: Bad DOI specified!
[84] Error: Bad DOI specified!
[85] Error: Bad DOI specified!
[86] Error: Bad DOI specified!
[87] "The GSF and FightSMA Announce 100K Research Award for the Development of a Large Animal Model of Spinal Muscular Atrophy" (http://www.fightsma.org/blog/uncategorized/the-gsf-and-fightsma-announce-100k-research-award). . Retrieved 18 December 2011.
[88] Error: Bad DOI specified!
[89] Error: Bad DOI specified!
[90] Error: Bad DOI specified!
[91] Error: Bad DOI specified!

Motor neurone disease

Amyotrophic lateral sclerosis

Classification and external resources

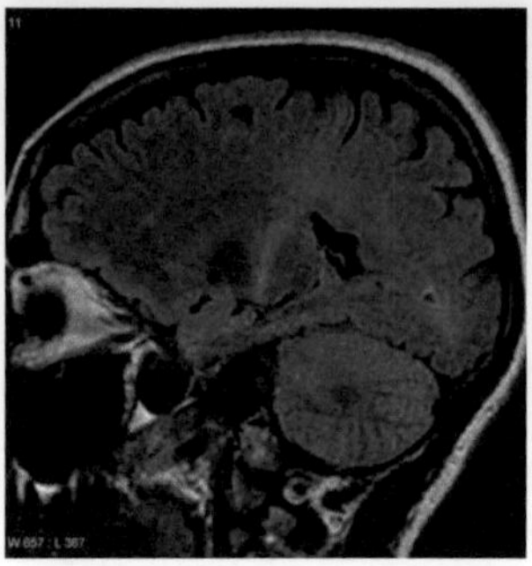

This MRI (parasagittal FLAIR) demonstrates increased T2 signal within the posterior part of the internal capsule and can be tracked to the subcortical white matter of the motor cortex, outlining the corticospinal tract, consistent with the clinical diagnosis of ALS. However, typically MRI imaging is unremarkable in a patient with ALS.

ICD-10	G12.2 [1]
ICD-9	335.20 [2]
OMIM	105400 [3]
DiseasesDB	29148 [4]
MedlinePlus	000688 [5]
eMedicine	neuro/14 [6] emerg/24 [7] pmr/10 [8]
MeSH	[17]

Amyotrophic lateral sclerosis (**ALS**) – also referred to as **motor neurone disease** in some Commonwealth of Nations countries and as **Lou Gehrig's disease** in the United States – is a debilitating disease with varied etiology characterized by rapidly progressive weakness, muscle atrophy and fasciculations, muscle spasticity, difficulty speaking (dysarthria), difficulty swallowing (dysphagia), and difficulty breathing (dyspnea). ALS is the most common of the five motor neuron diseases.

Signs and symptoms

The disorder causes muscle weakness and atrophy throughout the body caused by the degeneration of the upper and lower motor neurons. Unable to function, the muscles weaken and atrophy. Individuals affected by the disorder may ultimately lose the ability to initiate and control all voluntary movement, although bladder and bowel sphincters and the muscles responsible for eye movement are usually, but not always, spared until the terminal stages of the disease.[9]

Cognitive function is generally spared for most patients, although some (about 5%) also have frontotemporal dementia.[10] A higher proportion of patients (30–50%) also have more subtle cognitive changes which may go unnoticed, but are revealed by detailed neuropsychological testing. Sensory nerves and the autonomic nervous system are generally unaffected, meaning the majority of people with ALS will maintain hearing, sight, touch, smell, and taste.

Initial symptoms

The earliest symptoms of ALS are typically obvious weakness and/or muscle atrophy. Other presenting symptoms include muscle fasciculation (twitching), cramping, or stiffness of affected muscles; muscle weakness affecting an arm or a leg; and/or slurred and nasal speech. The parts of the body affected by early symptoms of ALS depend on which motor neurons in the body are damaged first. About 75% of people contracting the disease experience "limb onset" ALS, *i.e.*, first symptoms in the arms or legs. Patients with the leg onset form may experience awkwardness when walking or running or notice that they are tripping or stumbling, often with a "dropped foot" which drags gently along the ground. Arm-onset patients may experience difficulty with tasks requiring manual dexterity such as buttoning a shirt, writing, or turning a key in a lock. Occasionally, the symptoms remain confined to one limb for a long period of time or for the whole length of the illness; this is known as monomelic amyotrophy.

About 25% of cases are "bulbar onset" ALS. These patients first notice difficulty speaking clearly or swallowing. Speech may become slurred, nasal in character, or quieter. Other symptoms include difficulty swallowing and loss of tongue mobility. A smaller proportion of patients experience "respiratory onset" ALS, where the intercostal muscles that support breathing are affected first. A small proportion of patients may also present with what appears to be frontotemporal dementia, but later progresses to include more typical ALS symptoms.

Over time, patients experience increasing difficulty moving, swallowing (dysphagia), and speaking or forming words (dysarthria). Symptoms of upper motor neuron involvement include tight and stiff muscles (spasticity) and exaggerated reflexes (hyperreflexia) including an overactive gag reflex. An abnormal reflex commonly called Babinski's sign also indicates upper motor neuron damage. Symptoms of lower motor neuron degeneration include muscle weakness and atrophy, muscle cramps, and fleeting twitches of muscles that can be seen under the skin (fasciculations). Around 15–45% of patients experience pseudobulbar affect, also known as "emotional lability", which consists of uncontrollable laughter, crying or smiling, attributable to degeneration of bulbar upper motor neurons resulting in exaggeration of motor expressions of emotion. To be diagnosed with ALS, patients must have signs and symptoms of both upper and lower motor neuron damage that cannot be attributed to other causes.

Disease progression and spread

Although the order and rate of symptoms varies from person to person, eventually most patients are not able to walk, get out of bed on their own, or use their hands and arms. The rate of progression can be measured using an outcome measure called the "ALS Functional Rating Scale (Revised)", a 12-item instrument administered as a clinical interview or patient-reported questionnaire that produces a score between 48 (normal function) and 0 (severe disability). Though there is a high degree of variability and a small percentage of patients have much slower disease, on average, patients lose about 1 FRS point per month. Regardless of the part of the body first affected by the disease, muscle weakness and atrophy spread to other parts of the body as the disease progresses. In limb-onset ALS, symptoms usually spread from the affected limb to the opposite limb before affecting a new body region, whereas in bulbar-onset ALS symptoms typically spread to the arms before the legs.

Disease progression tends to be slower in patients who are younger than 40 at onset,[11] have disease restricted primarily to one limb, and those with primarily upper motor neuron symptoms.[12] Conversely, progression is faster and prognosis poorer in patients with bulbar-onset disease, respiratory-onset disease, and frontotemporal dementia.[12]

Late stage disease symptoms

Difficulty swallowing and chewing make eating normally very difficult and increase the risk of choking or aspirating food into the lungs. In later stages of the disease, aspiration pneumonia and maintaining a healthy weight can become a significant problem and may require insertion of a feeding tube. As the diaphragm and intercostal muscles (rib cage) that support breathing weaken, measures of lung function such as forced vital capacity and inspiratory pressure diminish. In respiratory onset ALS, this may occur before significant limb weakness is apparent. External machines such as bilevel positive pressure ventilation (frequently referred to by the tradename BiPAP) are frequently used to support breathing, first at night, and later during the daytime as well. BiPAP is only a temporary remedy, however, and it is recommended that long before BiPAP stops being effective, patients should decide whether to have a tracheotomy and long term mechanical ventilation. At this point, some patients choose palliative hospice care. Most people with ALS die of respiratory failure or pneumonia.

Although respiratory support can ease problems with breathing and prolong survival, it does not affect the progression of ALS. Most people with ALS die from respiratory failure, usually within three to five years from the onset of symptoms. The median survival time from onset to death is around 39 months, and only 4% survive longer than 10 years.[13] The best-known person with ALS, Stephen Hawking, has lived with the disease for more than 50 years, though his is an unusual case.[14]

Cause

Where no family history of the disease is present – i.e., in around 95% of cases – there is no known cause for ALS. Potential causes for which there is inconclusive evidence includes head trauma, military service, and participation in contact sports. Many other potential causes, including chemical exposure, electromagnetic field exposure, occupation, physical trauma, and electric shock, have been investigated but without consistent findings.[15]

According to Medical News Today, "A group of investigators from the University of British Columbia and the Vancouver Coastal Health Research Institute have discovered a crucial link between prions and the neurodegenerative disease ALS" [16]

There is a known hereditary factor in familial ALS (FALS), where the condition is known to run in families. Recently, a genetic abnormality known as a hexanucleotide repeat was found in a region called C9ORF72, which is associated with ALS combined with frontotemporal dementia ALS-FTD,[17] and accounts for some 6% of cases of ALS among white Europeans.[18] The high degree of mutations found in patients that appeared to have "sporadic" disease, *i.e.* without a family history, suggests that genetics may play a more significant role than previously thought and that environmental exposures may be less relevant.

A defect on chromosome 21 (coding for superoxide dismutase) is associated with approximately 20% of familial cases of ALS, or about 2% of ALS cases overall.[19] [20] [21] This mutation is believed to be autosomal dominant, and has over a hundred different forms of mutation. The most common ALS-causing SOD1 mutation in North American patients is A4V, characterized by an exceptionally rapid progression from onset to death. The most common mutation found in Scandinavian countries, D90A, is more slowly progressive than typical ALS and patients with this form of the disease survive for an average of 11 years.[22]

Mutations in several genes have also been linked to various types of ALS, and the currently identified associations are shown in the table below.

Type	OMIM	Gene	Locus	Remarks
ALS1	105400 [3]	*SOD1*	21q22.1	
ALS2	205100 [23]	*ALS2*	2q33.1	
ALS3	606640 [24]	?	18q21	
ALS4	602433 [25]	*SETX*	9q34.13	
ALS5	602099 [26]	?	15q15.1–q21.1	Juvenile onset
ALS6	608030 [27]	*FUS*	16p11.2	
ALS7	608031 [28]	?	20p13	
ALS8	608627 [29]	*VAPB*	20q13.3	
ALS9	611895 [30]	*ANG*	14q11.2	
ALS10	612069 [31]	*TARDBP*	1p36.2	
ALS11	612577 [32]	*FIG4*	6q21	
ALS12	613435 [33]	*OPTN*	10p13	
ALS13	183090 [34]	*ATXN2*	12q24.12	
ALS14	613954 [35]	*VCP*	9p13.3	Very rare, described only in one family[36]
ALS15	300857 [37]	*UBQLN2*	Xp11.23–p11.1	Described in one family[38]
ALS16	614373 [39]	*SIGMAR1*	9p13.3	Juvenile onset, very rare, described only in one family[40]
ALS17	614696 [41]	*CHMP2B*	3p11	Very rare, reported only in a handful of patients
ALS18	614808 [42]	*PFN1*	17p13.3	Very rare, described only in a handful of Chinese families[43]

Pathophysiology

The defining feature of ALS is the death of both upper and lower motor neurons in the motor cortex of the brain, the brain stem, and the spinal cord. Prior to their destruction, motor neurons develop proteinaceous inclusions in their cell bodies and axons. This may be partly due to defects in protein degradation.[44] These inclusions often contain ubiquitin, and generally incorporate one of the ALS-associated proteins: SOD1, TAR DNA binding protein (TDP-43, or TARDBP), or FUS.

SOD1

The cause of ALS is not known, though an important step toward determining the cause came in 1993 when scientists discovered that mutations in the gene that produces the Cu/Zn superoxide dismutase (SOD1) enzyme were associated with some cases (approximately 20%) of familial ALS. This enzyme is a powerful antioxidant that protects the body from damage caused by superoxide, a toxic free radical generated in the mitochondria. Free radicals are highly reactive molecules produced by cells during normal metabolism. Free radicals can accumulate and cause damage to both mitochondrial and nuclear DNA and proteins within cells. To date, over 110 different mutations in SOD1 have been linked with the disease, some of which have a very long clinical course (e.g. H46R), while others, such as A4V, being exceptionally aggressive. Evidence suggests that failure of defenses against oxidative stress up-regulates programmed cell death (apoptosis), among many other possible consequences.

Although it is not yet clear how the SOD1 gene mutation leads to motor neuron degeneration, researchers have theorized that an accumulation of free radicals may result from the faulty functioning of this gene. Current research, however, indicates that motor neuron death is not likely a result of lost or compromised dismutase activity, suggesting mutant SOD1 induces toxicity in some other way (a gain of function).[45] [46]

Studies involving transgenic mice have yielded several theories about the role of SOD1 in mutant SOD1 familial amyotrophic lateral sclerosis. Mice lacking the SOD1 gene entirely do not customarily develop ALS, although they do exhibit an acceleration of age-related muscle atrophy (sarcopenia) and a shortened lifespan (see article on superoxide dismutase). This indicates that the toxic properties of the mutant SOD1 are a result of a gain in function rather than a loss of normal function. In addition, aggregation of proteins has been found to be a common pathological feature of both familial and sporadic ALS (see article on proteopathy). Interestingly, in mutant SOD1 mice (most commonly, the G93A mutant), aggregates (misfolded protein accumulations) of mutant SOD1 were found only in diseased tissues, and greater amounts were detected during motor neuron degeneration.[47] It is speculated that aggregate accumulation of mutant SOD1 plays a role in disrupting cellular functions by damaging mitochondria, proteasomes, protein folding chaperones, or other proteins.[48] Any such disruption, if proven, would lend significant credibility to the theory that aggregates are involved in mutant SOD1 toxicity. Critics have noted that in humans, SOD1 mutations cause only 2% or so of overall cases and the etiological mechanisms may be distinct from those responsible for the sporadic form of the disease. To date, the ALS-SOD1 mice remain the best model of the disease for preclinical studies but it is hoped that more useful models will be developed.

Other factors

Studies also have focused on the role of glutamate in motor neuron degeneration. Glutamate is one of the chemical messengers or neurotransmitters in the brain. Scientists have found that, compared to healthy people, ALS patients have higher levels of glutamate in the serum and spinal fluid.[20] Riluzole is currently the only FDA approved drug for ALS and targets glutamate transporters. It only has a modest effect on survival, however, suggesting that excess glutamate is not the sole cause of the disease.

Diagnosis

No test can provide a definite diagnosis of ALS, although the presence of upper and lower motor neuron signs in a single limb is strongly suggestive. Instead, the diagnosis of ALS is primarily based on the symptoms and signs the physician observes in the patient and a series of tests to rule out other diseases. Physicians obtain the patient's full medical history and usually conduct a neurologic examination at regular intervals to assess whether symptoms such as muscle weakness, atrophy of muscles, hyperreflexia, and spasticity are getting progressively worse.

Because symptoms of ALS can be similar to those of a wide variety of other, more treatable diseases or disorders, appropriate tests must be conducted to exclude the possibility of other conditions. One of these tests is electromyography (EMG), a special recording technique that detects electrical activity in muscles. Certain EMG findings can support the diagnosis of ALS. Another common test measures nerve conduction velocity (NCV). Specific abnormalities in the NCV results may suggest, for example, that the patient has a form of peripheral neuropathy (damage to peripheral nerves) or myopathy (muscle disease) rather than ALS. The physician may order magnetic resonance imaging (MRI), a noninvasive procedure that uses a magnetic field and radio waves to take detailed images of the brain and spinal cord. Although these MRI scans are often normal in patients with ALS, they can reveal evidence of other problems that may be causing the symptoms, such as a spinal cord tumor, multiple sclerosis, a herniated disk in the neck, syringomyelia, or cervical spondylosis.

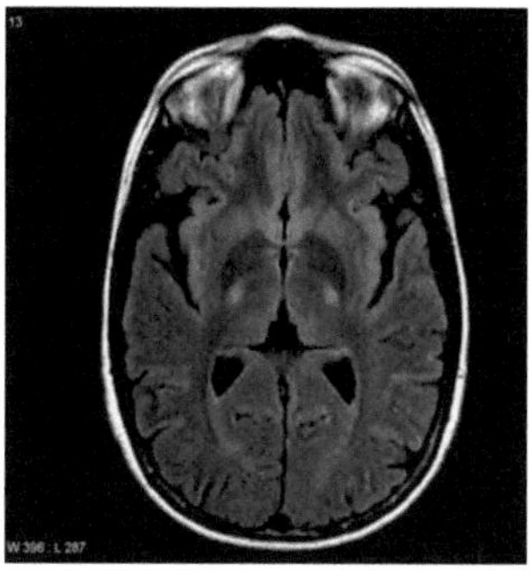

MRI (axial FLAIR) demonstrates increased T2 signal within the posterior part of the internal capsule, consistent with the clinical diagnosis of ALS.

Based on the patient's symptoms and findings from the examination and from these tests, the physician may order tests on blood and urine samples to eliminate the possibility of other diseases as well as routine laboratory tests. In some cases, for example, if a physician suspects that the patient may have a myopathy rather than ALS, a muscle biopsy may be performed.

Infectious diseases such as human immunodeficiency virus (HIV), human T-cell leukaemia virus (HTLV), Lyme disease,[49] syphilis[50] and tick-borne encephalitis[51] viruses can in some cases cause ALS-like symptoms. Neurological disorders such as multiple sclerosis, post-polio syndrome, multifocal motor neuropathy, CIDP, and spinal muscular atrophy can also mimic certain facets of the disease and should be considered by physicians attempting to make a diagnosis.

ALS must be differentiated from the "ALS mimic syndromes" which are unrelated disorders that may have a similar presentation and clinical features to ALS or its variants.[52] Because of the prognosis carried by this diagnosis and the variety of diseases or disorders that can resemble ALS in the early stages of the disease, patients should always obtain a second neurological opinion.

However, most cases of ALS are readily diagnosed and the error rate of diagnosis in large ALS clinics is less than 10%.[53] [54] In one study, 190 patients who met the MND / ALS diagnostic criteria, complemented with laboratory research in compliance with both research protocols and regular monitoring. Thirty of these patients (15.78%) had their diagnosis completely changed, during the clinical observation development period.[55] In the same study, three patients had a false negative diagnoses, myasthenia gravis (MG), an auto-immune disease. MG can mimic ALS and other neurological disorders leading to a delay in diagnosis and treatment. MG is eminently treatable; ALS is not.[56] Myasthenic syndrome, also known as Lambert-Eaton syndrome (LES),can mimic ALS and its initial presentation can be similar to that of MG.[57] [58]

Treatment

Slowing progression

Riluzole (Rilutek) is the only treatment that has been found to improve survival but only to a modest extent.[59] It lengthens survival by several months, and may have a greater survival benefit for those with a bulbar onset. It also extends the time before a person needs ventilation support. Riluzole does not reverse the damage already done to motor neurons, and people taking it must be monitored for liver damage (occurring in ~10% of people taking the drug).[60] It is approved by Food and Drug Administration (FDA) and recommended by the National Institute for Clinical Excellence (NICE).

Disease management

Other treatments for ALS are designed to relieve symptoms and improve the quality of life for patients. This supportive care is best provided by multidisciplinary teams of health care professionals working with patients and caregivers to keep patients as mobile and comfortable as possible.

Pharmaceutical treatments

Medical professionals can prescribe medications to help reduce fatigue, ease muscle cramps, control spasticity, and reduce excess saliva and phlegm. Drugs also are available to help patients with pain, depression, sleep disturbances, dysphagia, and constipation. Baclofen and diazepam are often prescribed to control the spasticity caused by ALS, and trihexyphenidyl or amitriptyline may be prescribed when ALS patients begin having trouble swallowing their saliva.[9]

Physical, occupational and speech therapy

Physical therapists and occupational therapists play a large role in rehabilitation for individuals with ALS. Specifically, physical and occupational therapists can set goals and promote benefits for individuals with ALS by delaying loss of strength, maintaining endurance, limiting pain, preventing complications, and promoting functional independence.[61]

Occupational therapy and special equipment such as assistive technology can also enhance patients' independence and safety throughout the course of ALS. Gentle, low-impact aerobic exercise such as performing activities of daily living (ADL's), walking, swimming, and stationary bicycling can strengthen unaffected muscles, improve cardiovascular health, and help patients fight fatigue and depression. Range of motion and stretching exercises can help prevent painful spasticity and shortening (contracture) of muscles. Physical and occupational therapists can recommend exercises that provide these benefits without overworking muscles. They can suggest devices such as ramps, braces, walkers, bathroom equipment (shower chairs, toilet risers, etc.) and wheelchairs that help patients remain mobile. Occupational therapists can provide or recommend equipment and adaptations to enable people to retain as much safety and independence in activities of daily living as possible.

ALS patients who have difficulty speaking may benefit from working with a speech-language pathologist. These health professionals can teach patients adaptive strategies such as techniques to help them speak louder and more clearly. As ALS progresses, speech-language pathologists can recommend the use of augmentative and alternative communication such as voice amplifiers, speech-generating devices (or voice output communication devices) and/or low tech communication techniques such as alphabet boards or yes/no signals.

Feeding and nutrition

Patients and caregivers can learn from speech-language pathologists and nutritionists how to plan and prepare numerous small meals throughout the day that provide enough calories, fiber, and fluid and how to avoid foods that are difficult to swallow. Patients may begin using suction devices to remove excess fluids or saliva and prevent choking. Occupational therapists can assist with recommendations for adaptive equipment to ease the physical task of self-feeding and/or make food choice recommendations that are more conducive to their unique deficits and abilities. When patients can no longer get enough nourishment from eating, doctors may advise inserting a feeding tube into the stomach. The use of a feeding tube also reduces the risk of choking and pneumonia that can result from inhaling liquids into the lungs. The tube is not painful and does not prevent patients from eating food orally if they wish.

Researchers have stated that "ALS patients have a chronically deficient intake of energy and recommended augmentation of energy intake."[62] Both animal[63] and human research[62] [64] suggest that ALS patients should be encouraged to consume as many calories as possible and not to restrict their calorie intake.

Breathing support

When the muscles that assist in breathing weaken, use of ventilatory assistance (intermittent positive pressure ventilation (IPPV), bilevel positive airway pressure (BIPAP), or biphasic cuirass ventilation (BCV)) may be used to aid breathing. Such devices artificially inflate the patient's lungs from various external sources that are applied directly to the face or body. When muscles are no longer able to maintain oxygen and carbon dioxide levels, these devices may be used full-time. BCV has the added advantage of being able to assist in clearing secretions by using high-frequency oscillations followed by several positive expiratory breaths.[65] Patients may eventually consider forms of mechanical ventilation (respirators) in which a machine inflates and deflates the lungs. To be effective, this may require a tube that passes from the nose or mouth to the windpipe (trachea) and for long-term use, an operation such as a tracheostomy, in which a plastic breathing tube is inserted directly in the patient's windpipe through an opening in the neck.

Patients and their families should consider several factors when deciding whether and when to use one of these options. Ventilation devices differ in their effect on the patient's quality of life and in cost. Although ventilation support can ease problems with breathing and prolong survival, it does not affect the progression of ALS. Patients need to be fully informed about these considerations and the long-term effects of life without movement before they make decisions about ventilation support. Some patients under long-term tracheostomy intermittent positive pressure ventilation with deflated cuffs or cuffless tracheostomy tubes (leak ventilation) are able to speak, provided their bulbar muscles are strong enough. This technique preserves speech in some patients with long-term mechanical ventilation. Other patients may be able to utilize a speaking valve such as a Passey-Muir Speaking Valve with the assistance and guidance of a speech-language pathologist.

Palliative care

Social workers and home care and hospice nurses help patients, families, and caregivers with the medical, emotional, and financial challenges of coping with ALS, particularly during the final stages of the disease. Social workers provide support such as assistance in obtaining financial aid, arranging durable power of attorney, preparing a living will, and finding support groups for patients and caregivers. Home nurses are available not only to provide medical care but also to teach caregivers about tasks such as maintaining respirators, giving feedings, and moving patients to avoid painful skin problems and contractures. Home hospice nurses work in consultation with physicians to ensure proper medication, pain control, and other care affecting the quality of life of patients who wish to remain at home. The home hospice team can also counsel patients and caregivers about end-of-life issues.

Epidemiology

ALS is one of the most common neuromuscular diseases worldwide, and people of all races and ethnic backgrounds are affected. One or two out of 100,000 people develop ALS each year.[66] ALS most commonly strikes people between 40 and 60 years of age, but younger and older people can also develop the disease. Men are affected slightly more often than women.

Although the incidence of ALS is thought to be regionally uniform, there are three regions in the West Pacific where there has in the past been an elevated occurrence of ALS. This seems to be declining in recent decades. The largest is the area of Guam inhabited by the Chamorro people, who have historically had a high incidence (as much as 143 cases per 100,000 people per year) of a condition called Lytico-Bodig disease which is a combination of symptoms similar to ALS, parkinsonism, and dementia. Lytico-Bodig disease has been linked to the consumption of cycad seeds and in particular, the chemical found in cycad seeds, β-methylamino-L-alanine (BMAA).[67] Two more areas of increased incidence are West Papua and the Kii Peninsula of Japan.[68] [69]

Although there have been reports of several "clusters" including three American football players from the San Francisco 49ers, more than fifty football players in Italy,[70] three football-playing friends in the south of England,[71] and reports of conjugal (husband and wife) cases in the south of France,[72] [73] [74] [75] [76] these are statistically plausible chance events. Although many authors consider ALS to be caused by a combination of genetic and environmental risk factors, so far the latter have not been firmly identified, other than a higher risk with increasing age.

Etymology

Amyotrophic comes from the Greek language: *A-* means "no", *myo* refers to "muscle", and *trophic* means "nourishment"; *amyotrophic* therefore means "no muscle nourishment," which describes the characteristic atrophication of the sufferer's disused muscle tissue. *Lateral* identifies the areas in a person's spinal cord where portions of the nerve cells that are affected are located. As this area degenerates it leads to scarring or hardening ("sclerosis") in the region.

History

Timeline

Year	Event
1824	Charles Bell writes a report about ALS.[77]
1850	English scientist Augustus Waller describes the appearance of shriveled nerve fibers
1869	French doctor Jean-Martin Charcot first describes ALS in scientific literature[78]
1881	"Amyotrophic Lateral Sclerosis" is translated into English and published in a three-volume edition of Lectures on the Diseases of the Nervous System
1939	ALS becomes a *cause célèbre* in the United States when baseball legend Lou Gehrig's career—and, two years later, his life—is ended by the disease. He gives his farewell speech on 4 July 1939.[79]
1950s	ALS epidemic occurs among the Chamorro people on Guam
1991	Researchers link chromosome 21 to FALS (Familial ALS)
1993	SOD1 gene on chromosome 21 found to play a role in some cases of FALS
1996	Rilutek becomes the first FDA-approved drug for ALS
1998	The El Escorial criteria is developed as the standard for classifying ALS patient in clinical research
1999	The revised ALS Functional Rating Scale (ALSFRS-R) is published and soon becomes a gold standard measure for rating decline in ALS patient in clinical research
2011	Noncoding repeat expansions in C9ORF72 are found to be a major cause of ALS and frontotemporal dementia

Clinical research

A number of clinical trials are underway globally for ALS; a comprehensive listing of trials in the US can be found at ClinicalTrials.gov.

Thalidomide and Lenalidomide have shown efficacy in protecting motor neurons in transgenic (G93A) mice.[80]

KNS-760704 (Dexpramipexole) is under clinical investigation in ALS patients. It is hoped that the drug will have a neuroprotective effect. It is one enantiomer of pramipexole, which is approved for the treatment of Parkinson's disease and restless legs syndrome.[81] The single-enantiomer preparation is essentially inactive at dopamine receptors, is not dose limited by the potent dopaminergic properties of pramipexole.[82] Results of a Phase II clinical trial conducted by Knopp Neurosciences and involving 102 patients were reported in 2010; the trial found a dose-dependent slowing in loss of function.[83] A larger phase II trial conducted by Biogen found the drug to be safe, well tolerated, and associated with a dose-dependent slowing in the decline of ALS.[84] In January 2013, Biogen Idec announced that it was discontinuing its development of dexpramipexole in ALS due to lack of efficacy in a Phase III study.

A Phase II trial on talampanel was completed by Teva Pharmaceutical Industries in April 2010 however it was found to be negative for treatment viability.[85]

See also

- ALS Association
- ALS Society of Canada
- ALS Therapy Development Institute
- Motor Neurone Disease Association
- Muscular Dystrophy Association

References

[1] http://apps.who.int/classifications/icd10/browse/2010/en#/G12.2
[2] http://www.icd9data.com/getICD9Code.ashx?icd9=335.20
[3] http://omim.org/entry/105400
[4] http://www.diseasesdatabase.com/ddb29148.htm
[5] http://www.nlm.nih.gov/medlineplus/ency/article/000688.htm
[6] http://www.emedicine.com/neuro/topic14.htm
[7] http://www.emedicine.com/emerg/topic24.htm#
[8] http://www.emedicine.com/pmr/topic10.htm#
[9] Dugdale DC, Hoch DB, Zieve D (August 27, 2010). "Amyotrophic lateral sclerosis" (http://www.ncbi.nlm.nih.gov/pubmedhealth/PMH0001708/). *A.D.A.M. Medical Encyclopedia.*.
[10] Phukan J, Pender NP, Hardiman O (2007). "Cognitive impairment in amyotrophic lateral sclerosis" (http://linkinghub.elsevier.com/retrieve/pii/S1474-4422(07)70265-X). *Lancet Neurol* **6** (11): 994–1003. doi:10.1016/S1474-4422(07)70265-X. PMID 17945153..
[11] Error: Bad DOI specified!
[12] Error: Bad DOI specified!
[13] Turner MR, Parton MJ, Shaw CE, Leigh PN, Al-Chalabi A (2003). "Prolonged survival in motor neuron disease: a descriptive study of the King's database 1990–2002.". *J Neurol Neurosurg Psychiatry* **74**: 995–997.
[14] "Stephen Hawking serves as role model for ALS patients" (http://articles.cnn.com/2009-04-20/health/hawking.als_1_als-association-lou-gehrig-s-disease-motor-neuron-disease?_s=PM:HEALTH). CNN. 2009-04-20..
[15] Sutedja NA, Fischer K, Veldink JH, van der Heijden GJ, Kromhout H, Heederik D, et al. (2009). "What we truly know about occupation as a risk factor for ALS: a critical and systematic review.". *Amyotrophic Lateral Sclerosis* **10**: 295–301.
[16] "Crucial Link Between Prions And ALS Discovered - May Transform Treatment" (http://www.medicalnewstoday.com/articles/234813.php). Medical News Today. 22 Sep 2011.. Retrieved 21 December 2012.
[17] Dejesus-Hernandez, M., et al., (2011). "Expanded GGGGCC Hexanucleotide Repeat in Noncoding Region of C9ORF72 Causes Chromosome 9p-Linked FTD and ALS.". *Neuron* **72** (2): 245–56.
[18] Majounie E., et al., (2012). "Frequency of the C9orf72 hexanucleotide repeat expansion in patients with amyotrophic lateral sclerosis and frontotemporal dementia: a cross-sectional study.". *Lancet Neurology* **11** (4): 323–330.

[19] Conwit, Robin A. (December 2006). "Preventing familial ALS: A clinical trial may be feasible but is an efficacy trial warranted?". *Journal of the Neurological Sciences* **251** (1–2): 1–2. doi:10.1016/j.jns.2006.07.009. ISSN 0022-510X. PMID 17070848.

[20] Al-Chalabi, Ammar; P. Nigel Leigh (August 2000). "Recent advances in amyotrophic lateral sclerosis". *Current Opinion in Neurology* **13** (4): 397–405. doi:10.1097/00019052-200008000-00006. ISSN 1473-6551. PMID 10970056.

[21] Battistini S, Ricci C, Lotti EM, Benigni M, Gagliardi S, Zucco R, Bondavalli M, Marcello N, Ceroni M, Cereda C (June 2010). "Severe familial ALS with a novel exon 4 mutation (L106F) in the SOD1 gene". *Journal of the Neurological Sciences* **293** (1): 112–115. doi:10.1016/j.jns.2010.03.009. PMID 20385392.

[22] Anderson P.M., et al., (1996). "Autosomal recessive adult-onset amyotrophic lateral sclerosis associated with homozygosity for Asp90Ala CuZn-superoxide dismutase mutation, A clinical and genealogical study of 36 patients.". *Brain* **119**: 1153–1172.

[23] http://omim.org/entry/205100

[24] http://omim.org/entry/606640

[25] http://omim.org/entry/602433

[26] http://omim.org/entry/602099

[27] http://omim.org/entry/608030

[28] http://omim.org/entry/608031

[29] http://omim.org/entry/608627

[30] http://omim.org/entry/611895

[31] http://omim.org/entry/612069

[32] http://omim.org/entry/612577

[33] http://omim.org/entry/613435

[34] http://omim.org/entry/183090

[35] http://omim.org/entry/613954

[36] Error: Bad DOI specified!

[37] http://omim.org/entry/300857

[38] Error: Bad DOI specified!

[39] http://omim.org/entry/614373

[40] Error: Bad DOI specified!

[41] http://omim.org/entry/614696

[42] http://omim.org/entry/614808

[43] Error: Bad DOI specified!

[44] Deng, HX; Chen, W, Hong, ST, Boycott, KM, Gorrie, GH, Siddique, N, Yang, Y, Fecto, F, Shi, Y, Zhai, H, Jiang, H, Hirano, M, Rampersaud, E, Jansen, GH, Donkervoort, S, Bigio, EH, Brooks, BR, Ajroud, K, Sufit, RL, Haines, JL, Mugnaini, E, Pericak-Vance, MA, Siddique, T (2011-08-21). "Mutations in UBQLN2 cause dominant X-linked juvenile and adult onset ALS and ALS/dementia". *Nature* **477** (7363): 211–5. doi:10.1038/nature10353. PMC 3169705. PMID 21857683.

[45] Reaume A, Elliott J, Hoffman E, Kowall N, Ferrante R, Siwek D, Wilcox H, Flood D, Beal M, Brown R, Scott R, Snider W (1996). "Motor neurons in Cu/Zn superoxide dismutase-deficient mice develop normally but exhibit enhanced cell death after axonal injury". *Nat Genet* **13** (1): 43–7. doi:10.1038/ng0596-43. PMID 8673102.

[46] Bruijn L, Houseweart M, Kato S, Anderson K, Anderson S, Ohama E, Reaume A, Scott R, Cleveland D (1998). "Aggregation and motor neuron toxicity of an ALS-linked SOD1 mutant independent from wild-type SOD1". *Science* **281** (5384): 1851–4. doi:10.1126/science.281.5384.1851. PMID 9743498.

[47] Furukawa Y, Fu R, Deng H, Siddique T, O'Halloran T (2006). "Disulfide cross-linked protein represents a significant fraction of ALS-associated Cu, Zn-superoxide dismutase aggregates in spinal cords of model mice". *Proc Natl Acad Sci USA* **103** (18): 7148–53. doi:10.1073/pnas.0602048103. PMC 1447524. PMID 16636274.

[48] Boillée S, Vande Velde C, Cleveland D (2006). "ALS: a disease of motor neurons and their nonneuronal neighbors". *Neuron* **52** (1): 39–59. doi:10.1016/j.neuron.2006.09.018. PMID 17015226.

[49] Hansel Y, Ackerl M, Stanek G. (1995). "ALS-like sequelae in chronic neuroborreliosis". *Wien Med Wochenschr.* **145** (7–8): 186–8. PMID 7610670.

[50] el Alaoui-Faris M, Medejel A, al Zemmouri K, Yahyaoui M, Chkili T (1990). "Amyotrophic lateral sclerosis syndrome of syphilitic origin. 5 cases". *Rev Neurol (Paris)* **146** (1): 41–4. PMID 2408129.

[51] Umanekii KG, Dekonenko EP (1983). "Structure of progressive forms of tick-borne encephalitis". *Zh Nevropatol Psikhiatr Im S S Korsakova.* **83** (8): 1173–9. PMID 6414202.

[52] Silani, V.; Messina, S.; Poletti, B.; Morelli, C.; Doretti, A.; Ticozzi, N.; Maderna, L. (2011). "The diagnosis of Amyotrophic lateral sclerosis in 2010". *Archives italiennes de biologie* **149** (1): 5–27. doi:10.4449/aib.v149i1.1260. PMID 21412713.

[53] Eisen, A. (2002). "Amyotrophic lateral sclerosis: A review" (http://www.bcmj.org/article/amyotrophic-lateral-sclerosis-review). *BCMJ* **44** (7): 362–366. .

[54] Error: Bad DOI specified!

[55] Error: Bad DOI specified!

[56] Al-Asmi, A.; Nandhagopal, R.; Jacob, P. C.; Gujjar, A. (2012). "Misdiagnosis of Myasthenia Gravis and Subsequent Clinical Implication: A case report and review of literature". *Sultan Qaboos University medical journal* **12** (1): 103–108. PMC 3286704. PMID 22375266.

[57] http://misc.medscape.com/pi/android/medscapeapp/html/A1170810-business.html

[58] http://www.lems.com/what_is_lems

[59] Carlesi, C; Pasquali, L, Piazza, S, Lo Gerfo, A, Caldarazzo Ienco, E, Alessi, R, Fornai, F, Siciliano, G (March 2011). "Strategies for clinical approach to neurodegeneration in Amyotrophic lateral sclerosis". *Archives italiennes de biologie* **149** (1): 151–67. doi:10.4449/aib.v149i1.1267. PMID 21412722.

[60] Miller, RG; Mitchell JD, Lyon M, Moore DH, G (2007). Miller, Robert G. ed. "Riluzole for amyotrophic lateral sclerosis (ALS)/motor neuron disease (MND)". *Cochrane Database of Systematic Reviews* (1): CD001447. doi:10.1002/14651858.CD001447.pub2. PMID 17253460.

[61] Lewis, M. & Rushanan, S. (2007). "The role of physical therapy and occupational therapy in the treatment of Amyotrophic Lateral Sclerosis". *NeuroRehabilitation* **22** (6): 451–461. PMID 18198431.

[62] Kasarskis EJ, Berryman S, Vanderleest JG, Schneider AR, McClain CJ (Jan 1996). "Nutritional status of patients with amyotrophic lateral sclerosis: relation to the proximity of death" (http://www.ajcn.org/cgi/pmidlookup?view=long&pmid=8604660). *Am J Clin Nutr.* **63** (1): 130–7. PMID 8604660. .

[63] Hamadeh MJ, Rodriguez MC, Kaczor JJ, Tarnopolsky MA (Feb 2005). "Caloric restriction transiently improves motor performance but hastens clinical onset of disease in the Cu/Zn-superoxide dismutase mutant G93A mouse". *Muscle Nerve* **31** (2): 214–20. doi:10.1002/mus.20255. PMID 15625688.

[64] Slowie LA, Paige MS, Antel JP (Jul 1983). "Nutritional considerations in the management of patients with amyotrophic lateral sclerosis (ALS)". *J Am Diet Assoc* **83** (1): 44–7. PMID 6863783.

[65] Sviri S, Linton DM, Van Heerden PV (Jun 2005). "Non-invasive Mechanical Ventilation Enhances Patient Autonomy in Decision-Making Regarding Chronic Ventilation". *Critical Care and Resuscitation* **7** (2): 116–118. PMID 16548804.

[66] "ALS Topic Overview" (http://www.webmd.com/brain/tc/Amyotrophic-Lateral-Sclerosis-ALS-Topic-Overview). Archived (http://web.archive.org/web/20080501194730/http://www.webmd.com/brain/tc/amyotrophic-lateral-sclerosis-als-topic-overview) from the original on 1 May 2008. . Retrieved 2008-05-01.

[67] Reed D, Labarthe D, Chen KM, Stallones R (Jan 1987). "A cohort study of amyotrophic lateral sclerosis and parkinsonism-dementia on Guam and Rota" (http://aje.oxfordjournals.org/cgi/pmidlookup?view=long&pmid=3788958). *Am J Epidemiol.* **125** (1): 92–100. PMID 3788958. .

[68] S. Kuzuhara, Y. Kokubo P3-146Marked increase of parkinsonism-dementia (P-D) phenotypes in the high incidence amyotrophic lateral sclerosis (ALS) focus in the Kii peninsula of Japan. Alzheimer's and Dementia, Volume 2, Issue 3, Pages S417-S417

[69] Spencer PS, Palmer VS, Ludolph AC (Aug 2005). "On the decline and etiology of high-incidence motor system disease in West Papua (southwest New Guinea)". *Mov. Disord.* **20** (Suppl 12): S119–26. doi:10.1002/mds.20552. PMID 16092101.

[70] "Sla, indagini nei club. Pesticidi nel mirino" (http://www.corriere.it/sport/08_ottobre_03/sla_indagine_pesticidi_fd04f986-911c-11dd-9f28-00144f02aabc.shtml). Archived (http://web.archive.org/web/20081003220654/http://www.corriere.it/sport/08_ottobre_03/sla_indagine_pesticidi_fd04f986-911c-11dd-9f28-00144f02aabc.shtml) from the original on 3 October 2008. . Retrieved 2008-10-02.

[71] Wicks P, Abrahams S, Masi D, Hejda-Forde S, Leigh PN & Goldstein LH (2005) The Prevalence of Depression and Anxiety in MND, Amyotrophic Lateral Sclerosis and other Motor Neuron Disorders, Volume 6, Supplement 1, p. 147

[72] Rachele MG, Mascia V, Tacconi P, Dessi N, Marrosu F (April 1998). "Conjugal amyotrophic lateral sclerosis: a report on a couple from Sardinia, Italy". *Ital J Neurol Sci.* **19** (2): 97–100. doi:10.1007/BF02427565. PMID 10935845.

[73] Poloni M, Micheli A, Facchetti D, Mai R, Ceriani F (April 1997). "Conjugal amyotrophic lateral sclerosis: toxic clustering or change?". *Ital J Neurol Sci.* **18** (2): 109–12. doi:10.1007/BF01999572. PMID 9239532.

[74] Camu W, Cadilhac J, Billiard M. (March 1994). "Conjugal amyotrophic lateral sclerosis: a report on two couples from southern France". *Neurology* **44** (3 Pt 1): 547–8. PMID 8145930.

[75] Cornblath DR, Kurland LT, Boylan KB, Morrison L, Radhakrishnan K, Montgomery M. (November 1993). "Conjugal amyotrophic lateral sclerosis: report of a young married couple". *Neurology* **43** (11): 2378–80. PMID 8232960.

[76] Corcia P, Jafari-Schluep HF, Lardillier D, Mazyad H, Giraud P, Clavelou P, Pouget J, Camu W (November 2003). "A clustering of conjugal amyotrophic lateral sclerosis in southeastern France". *Neurol.* **60** (4): 553–7. doi:10.1001/archneur.60.4.553. PMID 12707069.

[77] Tyler HR, Shefner J. Amyotrophic lateral sclerosis. Handb Clin Neurol. 1991;15:169–215. Serial publication.

[78] Rowland LP (March 2001). "How amyotrophic lateral sclerosis got its name: the clinical-pathologic genius of Jean-Martin Charcot" (http://archneur.ama-assn.org/cgi/content/extract/58/3/512). *Arch. Neurol.* **58** (3): 512–5. doi:10.1001/archneur.58.3.512. PMID 11255459. .

[79] "Farewell Speech" (http://www.lougehrig.com/about/speech.htm). lougehrig.com. 4 July 1939. Archived (http://web.archive.org/web/20080412123358/http://www.lougehrig.com/about/speech.htm) from the original on 12 April 2008. . Retrieved 16 April 2008.

[80] *The Journal of Neuroscience* **26** (9): 2467-2473. March 1 2006. http://www.jneurosci.org/content/26/9/2467.full.pdf+html.

[81] Abramova NA et al. (2002 Feb 15). "Inhibition by R(+) or S(-) pramipexole of caspase activation and cell death induced by methylpyridinium ion or beta amyloid peptide in SH-SY5Y neuroblastoma". *J Neurosci Res* **67** (4): 494–500. PMID 11835316.

[82] Error: Bad DOI specified!

[83] Error: Bad DOI specified!

[84] Error: Bad DOI specified!

[85] "Talampanel for Amyotrophic Lateral Sclerosis (ALS)". ClinicalTrials.gov.

Further reading

- "ALS Hope Foundation" (http://www.alshopefoundation.org/). Archived (http://web.archive.org/web/20080512012521/http://www.alshopefoundation.org/) from the original on 12 May 2008. Retrieved 2008-06-21. "Dedicated to the care and cure of people with Lou Gehrig's Disease. (from site page us.php)"
- "Lou Gehrig: The Official Web Site" (http://www.lougehrig.com). CMG Worldwide. Archived (http://web.archive.org/web/20080509101328/http://www.lougehrig.com/) from the original on 9 May 2008. Retrieved 2008-06-21. "The Official Web site of Lou Gehrig is an informational Web site intended to honor the life, the legend and the career of Lou Gehrig. (from site page siteinfo/index.htm)"
- Patrick Aebischer; Ann C. Kato (November 2007). "Playing defense against Lou Gehrig's Disease" (http://www.sciam.com/article.cfm?id=playing-defense-against-l) (Paper). *Scientific American* (Verlagsgruppe Georg von Holtzbrinck): pp. 86–93. Retrieved 2008-06-21. "Researchers have proposed potential therapies for a paralyzing disorder once thought to be untreatable (sub-title)"

External links

- Medline Plus article on ALS (https://www.nlm.nih.gov/medlineplus/amyotrophiclateralsclerosis.html)

Motor neurone disease

Amyotrophic lateral sclerosis	
Classification and external resources	

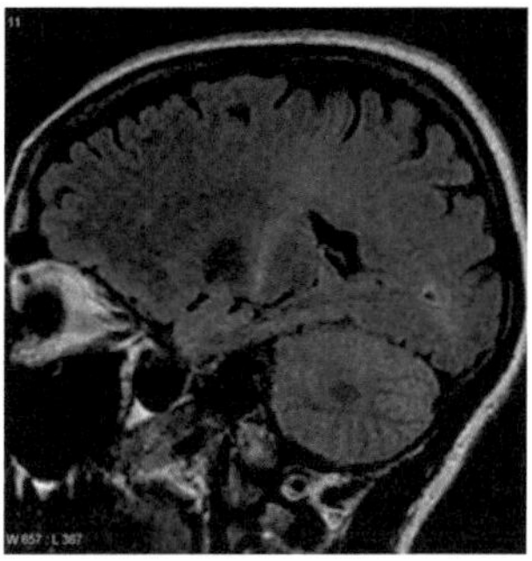

This MRI (parasagittal FLAIR) demonstrates increased T2 signal within the posterior part of the internal capsule and can be tracked to the subcortical white matter of the motor cortex, outlining the corticospinal tract, consistent with the clinical diagnosis of ALS. However, typically MRI imaging is unremarkable in a patient with ALS.

ICD-10	G12.2 [1]
ICD-9	335.20 [2]
OMIM	105400 [3]
DiseasesDB	29148 [4]
MedlinePlus	000688 [5]
eMedicine	neuro/14 [6] emerg/24 [7] pmr/10 [8]
MeSH	[17]

Amyotrophic lateral sclerosis (**ALS**) – also referred to as **motor neurone disease** in some Commonwealth of Nations countries and as **Lou Gehrig's disease** in the United States – is a debilitating disease with varied etiology characterized by rapidly progressive weakness, muscle atrophy and fasciculations, muscle spasticity, difficulty speaking (dysarthria), difficulty swallowing (dysphagia), and difficulty breathing (dyspnea). ALS is the most common of the five motor neuron diseases.

Signs and symptoms

The disorder causes muscle weakness and atrophy throughout the body caused by the degeneration of the upper and lower motor neurons. Unable to function, the muscles weaken and atrophy. Individuals affected by the disorder may ultimately lose the ability to initiate and control all voluntary movement, although bladder and bowel sphincters and the muscles responsible for eye movement are usually, but not always, spared until the terminal stages of the disease.[1]

Cognitive function is generally spared for most patients, although some (about 5%) also have frontotemporal dementia.[2] A higher proportion of patients (30–50%) also have more subtle cognitive changes which may go unnoticed, but are revealed by detailed neuropsychological testing. Sensory nerves and the autonomic nervous system are generally unaffected, meaning the majority of people with ALS will maintain hearing, sight, touch, smell, and taste.

Initial symptoms

The earliest symptoms of ALS are typically obvious weakness and/or muscle atrophy. Other presenting symptoms include muscle fasciculation (twitching), cramping, or stiffness of affected muscles; muscle weakness affecting an arm or a leg; and/or slurred and nasal speech. The parts of the body affected by early symptoms of ALS depend on which motor neurons in the body are damaged first. About 75% of people contracting the disease experience "limb onset" ALS, *i.e.*, first symptoms in the arms or legs. Patients with the leg onset form may experience awkwardness when walking or running or notice that they are tripping or stumbling, often with a "dropped foot" which drags gently along the ground. Arm-onset patients may experience difficulty with tasks requiring manual dexterity such as buttoning a shirt, writing, or turning a key in a lock. Occasionally, the symptoms remain confined to one limb for a long period of time or for the whole length of the illness; this is known as monomelic amyotrophy.

About 25% of cases are "bulbar onset" ALS. These patients first notice difficulty speaking clearly or swallowing. Speech may become slurred, nasal in character, or quieter. Other symptoms include difficulty swallowing and loss of tongue mobility. A smaller proportion of patients experience "respiratory onset" ALS, where the intercostal muscles that support breathing are affected first. A small proportion of patients may also present with what appears to be frontotemporal dementia, but later progresses to include more typical ALS symptoms.

Over time, patients experience increasing difficulty moving, swallowing (dysphagia), and speaking or forming words (dysarthria). Symptoms of upper motor neuron involvement include tight and stiff muscles (spasticity) and exaggerated reflexes (hyperreflexia) including an overactive gag reflex. An abnormal reflex commonly called Babinski's sign also indicates upper motor neuron damage. Symptoms of lower motor neuron degeneration include muscle weakness and atrophy, muscle cramps, and fleeting twitches of muscles that can be seen under the skin (fasciculations). Around 15–45% of patients experience pseudobulbar affect, also known as "emotional lability", which consists of uncontrollable laughter, crying or smiling, attributable to degeneration of bulbar upper motor neurons resulting in exaggeration of motor expressions of emotion. To be diagnosed with ALS, patients must have signs and symptoms of both upper and lower motor neuron damage that cannot be attributed to other causes.

Disease progression and spread

Although the order and rate of symptoms varies from person to person, eventually most patients are not able to walk, get out of bed on their own, or use their hands and arms. The rate of progression can be measured using an outcome measure called the "ALS Functional Rating Scale (Revised)", a 12-item instrument administered as a clinical interview or patient-reported questionnaire that produces a score between 48 (normal function) and 0 (severe disability). Though there is a high degree of variability and a small percentage of patients have much slower disease, on average, patients lose about 1 FRS point per month. Regardless of the part of the body first affected by the disease, muscle weakness and atrophy spread to other parts of the body as the disease progresses. In limb-onset ALS, symptoms usually spread from the affected limb to the opposite limb before affecting a new body region, whereas in bulbar-onset ALS symptoms typically spread to the arms before the legs.

Disease progression tends to be slower in patients who are younger than 40 at onset,[3] have disease restricted primarily to one limb, and those with primarily upper motor neuron symptoms.[4] Conversely, progression is faster and prognosis poorer in patients with bulbar-onset disease, respiratory-onset disease, and frontotemporal dementia.[4]

Late stage disease symptoms

Difficulty swallowing and chewing make eating normally very difficult and increase the risk of choking or aspirating food into the lungs. In later stages of the disease, aspiration pneumonia and maintaining a healthy weight can become a significant problem and may require insertion of a feeding tube. As the diaphragm and intercostal muscles (rib cage) that support breathing weaken, measures of lung function such as forced vital capacity and inspiratory pressure diminish. In respiratory onset ALS, this may occur before significant limb weakness is apparent. External machines such as bilevel positive pressure ventilation (frequently referred to by the tradename BiPAP) are frequently used to support breathing, first at night, and later during the daytime as well. BiPAP is only a temporary remedy, however, and it is recommended that long before BiPAP stops being effective, patients should decide whether to have a tracheotomy and long term mechanical ventilation. At this point, some patients choose palliative hospice care. Most people with ALS die of respiratory failure or pneumonia.

Although respiratory support can ease problems with breathing and prolong survival, it does not affect the progression of ALS. Most people with ALS die from respiratory failure, usually within three to five years from the onset of symptoms. The median survival time from onset to death is around 39 months, and only 4% survive longer than 10 years.[5] The best-known person with ALS, Stephen Hawking, has lived with the disease for more than 50 years, though his is an unusual case.[6]

Cause

Where no family history of the disease is present – i.e., in around 95% of cases – there is no known cause for ALS. Potential causes for which there is inconclusive evidence includes head trauma, military service, and participation in contact sports. Many other potential causes, including chemical exposure, electromagnetic field exposure, occupation, physical trauma, and electric shock, have been investigated but without consistent findings.[7]

According to Medical News Today, "A group of investigators from the University of British Columbia and the Vancouver Coastal Health Research Institute have discovered a crucial link between prions and the neurodegenerative disease ALS" [8]

There is a known hereditary factor in familial ALS (FALS), where the condition is known to run in families. Recently, a genetic abnormality known as a hexanucleotide repeat was found in a region called C9ORF72, which is associated with ALS combined with frontotemporal dementia ALS-FTD,[9] and accounts for some 6% of cases of ALS among white Europeans.[10] The high degree of mutations found in patients that appeared to have "sporadic" disease, *i.e.* without a family history, suggests that genetics may play a more significant role than previously thought and that environmental exposures may be less relevant.

A defect on chromosome 21 (coding for superoxide dismutase) is associated with approximately 20% of familial cases of ALS, or about 2% of ALS cases overall.[11] [12] [13] This mutation is believed to be autosomal dominant, and has over a hundred different forms of mutation. The most common ALS-causing SOD1 mutation in North American patients is A4V, characterized by an exceptionally rapid progression from onset to death. The most common mutation found in Scandinavian countries, D90A, is more slowly progressive than typical ALS and patients with this form of the disease survive for an average of 11 years.[14]

Mutations in several genes have also been linked to various types of ALS, and the currently identified associations are shown in the table below.

Type	OMIM	Gene	Locus	Remarks
ALS1	105400 [3]	*SOD1*	21q22.1	
ALS2	205100 [23]	*ALS2*	2q33.1	
ALS3	606640 [24]	?	18q21	
ALS4	602433 [25]	*SETX*	9q34.13	
ALS5	602099 [26]	?	15q15.1–q21.1	Juvenile onset
ALS6	608030 [27]	*FUS*	16p11.2	
ALS7	608031 [28]	?	20p13	
ALS8	608627 [29]	*VAPB*	20q13.3	
ALS9	611895 [30]	*ANG*	14q11.2	
ALS10	612069 [31]	*TARDBP*	1p36.2	
ALS11	612577 [32]	*FIG4*	6q21	
ALS12	613435 [33]	*OPTN*	10p13	
ALS13	183090 [34]	*ATXN2*	12q24.12	
ALS14	613954 [35]	*VCP*	9p13.3	Very rare, described only in one family[15]
ALS15	300857 [37]	*UBQLN2*	Xp11.23–p11.1	Described in one family[16]
ALS16	614373 [39]	*SIGMAR1*	9p13.3	Juvenile onset, very rare, described only in one family[17]
ALS17	614696 [41]	*CHMP2B*	3p11	Very rare, reported only in a handful of patients
ALS18	614808 [42]	*PFN1*	17p13.3	Very rare, described only in a handful of Chinese families[18]

Pathophysiology

The defining feature of ALS is the death of both upper and lower motor neurons in the motor cortex of the brain, the brain stem, and the spinal cord. Prior to their destruction, motor neurons develop proteinaceous inclusions in their cell bodies and axons. This may be partly due to defects in protein degradation.[19] These inclusions often contain ubiquitin, and generally incorporate one of the ALS-associated proteins: SOD1, TAR DNA binding protein (TDP-43, or TARDBP), or FUS.

SOD1

The cause of ALS is not known, though an important step toward determining the cause came in 1993 when scientists discovered that mutations in the gene that produces the Cu/Zn superoxide dismutase (SOD1) enzyme were associated with some cases (approximately 20%) of familial ALS. This enzyme is a powerful antioxidant that protects the body from damage caused by superoxide, a toxic free radical generated in the mitochondria. Free radicals are highly reactive molecules produced by cells during normal metabolism. Free radicals can accumulate and cause damage to both mitochondrial and nuclear DNA and proteins within cells. To date, over 110 different mutations in SOD1 have been linked with the disease, some of which have a very long clinical course (e.g. H46R), while others, such as A4V, being exceptionally aggressive. Evidence suggests that failure of defenses against oxidative stress up-regulates programmed cell death (apoptosis), among many other possible consequences.

Although it is not yet clear how the SOD1 gene mutation leads to motor neuron degeneration, researchers have theorized that an accumulation of free radicals may result from the faulty functioning of this gene. Current research, however, indicates that motor neuron death is not likely a result of lost or compromised dismutase activity, suggesting mutant SOD1 induces toxicity in some other way (a gain of function).[20] [21]

Studies involving transgenic mice have yielded several theories about the role of SOD1 in mutant SOD1 familial amyotrophic lateral sclerosis. Mice lacking the SOD1 gene entirely do not customarily develop ALS, although they do exhibit an acceleration of age-related muscle atrophy (sarcopenia) and a shortened lifespan (see article on superoxide dismutase). This indicates that the toxic properties of the mutant SOD1 are a result of a gain in function rather than a loss of normal function. In addition, aggregation of proteins has been found to be a common pathological feature of both familial and sporadic ALS (see article on proteopathy). Interestingly, in mutant SOD1 mice (most commonly, the G93A mutant), aggregates (misfolded protein accumulations) of mutant SOD1 were found only in diseased tissues, and greater amounts were detected during motor neuron degeneration.[22] It is speculated that aggregate accumulation of mutant SOD1 plays a role in disrupting cellular functions by damaging mitochondria, proteasomes, protein folding chaperones, or other proteins.[23] Any such disruption, if proven, would lend significant credibility to the theory that aggregates are involved in mutant SOD1 toxicity. Critics have noted that in humans, SOD1 mutations cause only 2% or so of overall cases and the etiological mechanisms may be distinct from those responsible for the sporadic form of the disease. To date, the ALS-SOD1 mice remain the best model of the disease for preclinical studies but it is hoped that more useful models will be developed.

Other factors

Studies also have focused on the role of glutamate in motor neuron degeneration. Glutamate is one of the chemical messengers or neurotransmitters in the brain. Scientists have found that, compared to healthy people, ALS patients have higher levels of glutamate in the serum and spinal fluid.[12] Riluzole is currently the only FDA approved drug for ALS and targets glutamate transporters. It only has a modest effect on survival, however, suggesting that excess glutamate is not the sole cause of the disease.

Diagnosis

No test can provide a definite diagnosis of ALS, although the presence of upper and lower motor neuron signs in a single limb is strongly suggestive. Instead, the diagnosis of ALS is primarily based on the symptoms and signs the physician observes in the patient and a series of tests to rule out other diseases. Physicians obtain the patient's full medical history and usually conduct a neurologic examination at regular intervals to assess whether symptoms such as muscle weakness, atrophy of muscles, hyperreflexia, and spasticity are getting progressively worse.

Because symptoms of ALS can be similar to those of a wide variety of other, more treatable diseases or disorders, appropriate tests must be conducted to exclude the possibility of other conditions. One of these tests is electromyography (EMG), a special recording technique that detects electrical activity in muscles. Certain EMG findings can support the diagnosis of ALS. Another common test measures nerve conduction velocity (NCV). Specific abnormalities in the NCV results may suggest, for example, that the patient has a form of peripheral neuropathy (damage to peripheral nerves) or myopathy (muscle disease) rather than ALS. The physician may order magnetic resonance imaging (MRI), a noninvasive procedure that uses a magnetic field and radio waves to take detailed images of the brain and spinal cord. Although these MRI scans are often normal in patients with ALS, they can reveal evidence of other problems that may be causing the symptoms, such as a spinal cord tumor, multiple sclerosis, a herniated disk in the neck, syringomyelia, or cervical spondylosis.

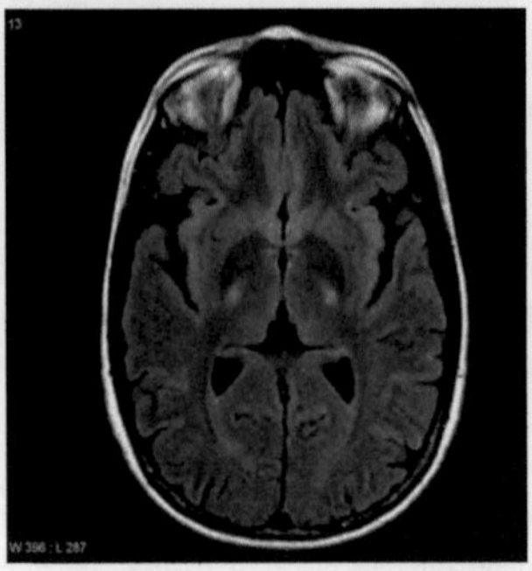

MRI (axial FLAIR) demonstrates increased T2 signal within the posterior part of the internal capsule, consistent with the clinical diagnosis of ALS.

Based on the patient's symptoms and findings from the examination and from these tests, the physician may order tests on blood and urine samples to eliminate the possibility of other diseases as well as routine laboratory tests. In some cases, for example, if a physician suspects that the patient may have a myopathy rather than ALS, a muscle biopsy may be performed.

Infectious diseases such as human immunodeficiency virus (HIV), human T-cell leukaemia virus (HTLV), Lyme disease,[24] syphilis[25] and tick-borne encephalitis[26] viruses can in some cases cause ALS-like symptoms. Neurological disorders such as multiple sclerosis, post-polio syndrome, multifocal motor neuropathy, CIDP, and spinal muscular atrophy can also mimic certain facets of the disease and should be considered by physicians attempting to make a diagnosis.

ALS must be differentiated from the "ALS mimic syndromes" which are unrelated disorders that may have a similar presentation and clinical features to ALS or its variants.[27] Because of the prognosis carried by this diagnosis and the variety of diseases or disorders that can resemble ALS in the early stages of the disease, patients should always obtain a second neurological opinion.

However, most cases of ALS are readily diagnosed and the error rate of diagnosis in large ALS clinics is less than 10%.[28] [29] In one study, 190 patients who met the MND / ALS diagnostic criteria, complemented with laboratory research in compliance with both research protocols and regular monitoring. Thirty of these patients (15.78%) had their diagnosis completely changed, during the clinical observation development period.[30] In the same study, three patients had a false negative diagnoses, myasthenia gravis (MG), an auto-immune disease. MG can mimic ALS and other neurological disorders leading to a delay in diagnosis and treatment. MG is eminently treatable; ALS is not.[31] Myasthenic syndrome, also known as Lambert-Eaton syndrome (LES),can mimic ALS and its initial presentation can be similar to that of MG.[32] [33]

Treatment

Slowing progression

Riluzole (Rilutek) is the only treatment that has been found to improve survival but only to a modest extent.[34] It lengthens survival by several months, and may have a greater survival benefit for those with a bulbar onset. It also extends the time before a person needs ventilation support. Riluzole does not reverse the damage already done to motor neurons, and people taking it must be monitored for liver damage (occurring in ~10% of people taking the drug).[35] It is approved by Food and Drug Administration (FDA) and recommended by the National Institute for Clinical Excellence (NICE).

Disease management

Other treatments for ALS are designed to relieve symptoms and improve the quality of life for patients. This supportive care is best provided by multidisciplinary teams of health care professionals working with patients and caregivers to keep patients as mobile and comfortable as possible.

Pharmaceutical treatments

Medical professionals can prescribe medications to help reduce fatigue, ease muscle cramps, control spasticity, and reduce excess saliva and phlegm. Drugs also are available to help patients with pain, depression, sleep disturbances, dysphagia, and constipation. Baclofen and diazepam are often prescribed to control the spasticity caused by ALS, and trihexyphenidyl or amitriptyline may be prescribed when ALS patients begin having trouble swallowing their saliva.[1]

Physical, occupational and speech therapy

Physical therapists and occupational therapists play a large role in rehabilitation for individuals with ALS. Specifically, physical and occupational therapists can set goals and promote benefits for individuals with ALS by delaying loss of strength, maintaining endurance, limiting pain, preventing complications, and promoting functional independence.[36]

Occupational therapy and special equipment such as assistive technology can also enhance patients' independence and safety throughout the course of ALS. Gentle, low-impact aerobic exercise such as performing activities of daily living (ADL's), walking, swimming, and stationary bicycling can strengthen unaffected muscles, improve cardiovascular health, and help patients fight fatigue and depression. Range of motion and stretching exercises can help prevent painful spasticity and shortening (contracture) of muscles. Physical and occupational therapists can recommend exercises that provide these benefits without overworking muscles. They can suggest devices such as ramps, braces, walkers, bathroom equipment (shower chairs, toilet risers, etc.) and wheelchairs that help patients remain mobile. Occupational therapists can provide or recommend equipment and adaptations to enable people to retain as much safety and independence in activities of daily living as possible.

ALS patients who have difficulty speaking may benefit from working with a speech-language pathologist. These health professionals can teach patients adaptive strategies such as techniques to help them speak louder and more clearly. As ALS progresses, speech-language pathologists can recommend the use of augmentative and alternative communication such as voice amplifiers, speech-generating devices (or voice output communication devices) and/or low tech communication techniques such as alphabet boards or yes/no signals.

Feeding and nutrition

Patients and caregivers can learn from speech-language pathologists and nutritionists how to plan and prepare numerous small meals throughout the day that provide enough calories, fiber, and fluid and how to avoid foods that are difficult to swallow. Patients may begin using suction devices to remove excess fluids or saliva and prevent choking. Occupational therapists can assist with recommendations for adaptive equipment to ease the physical task of self-feeding and/or make food choice recommendations that are more conducive to their unique deficits and abilities. When patients can no longer get enough nourishment from eating, doctors may advise inserting a feeding tube into the stomach. The use of a feeding tube also reduces the risk of choking and pneumonia that can result from inhaling liquids into the lungs. The tube is not painful and does not prevent patients from eating food orally if they wish.

Researchers have stated that "ALS patients have a chronically deficient intake of energy and recommended augmentation of energy intake."[37] Both animal[38] and human research[37] [39] suggest that ALS patients should be encouraged to consume as many calories as possible and not to restrict their calorie intake.

Breathing support

When the muscles that assist in breathing weaken, use of ventilatory assistance (intermittent positive pressure ventilation (IPPV), bilevel positive airway pressure (BIPAP), or biphasic cuirass ventilation (BCV)) may be used to aid breathing. Such devices artificially inflate the patient's lungs from various external sources that are applied directly to the face or body. When muscles are no longer able to maintain oxygen and carbon dioxide levels, these devices may be used full-time. BCV has the added advantage of being able to assist in clearing secretions by using high-frequency oscillations followed by several positive expiratory breaths.[40] Patients may eventually consider forms of mechanical ventilation (respirators) in which a machine inflates and deflates the lungs. To be effective, this may require a tube that passes from the nose or mouth to the windpipe (trachea) and for long-term use, an operation such as a tracheostomy, in which a plastic breathing tube is inserted directly in the patient's windpipe through an opening in the neck.

Patients and their families should consider several factors when deciding whether and when to use one of these options. Ventilation devices differ in their effect on the patient's quality of life and in cost. Although ventilation support can ease problems with breathing and prolong survival, it does not affect the progression of ALS. Patients need to be fully informed about these considerations and the long-term effects of life without movement before they make decisions about ventilation support. Some patients under long-term tracheostomy intermittent positive pressure ventilation with deflated cuffs or cuffless tracheostomy tubes (leak ventilation) are able to speak, provided their bulbar muscles are strong enough. This technique preserves speech in some patients with long-term mechanical ventilation. Other patients may be able to utilize a speaking valve such as a Passey-Muir Speaking Valve with the assistance and guidance of a speech-language pathologist.

Palliative care

Social workers and home care and hospice nurses help patients, families, and caregivers with the medical, emotional, and financial challenges of coping with ALS, particularly during the final stages of the disease. Social workers provide support such as assistance in obtaining financial aid, arranging durable power of attorney, preparing a living will, and finding support groups for patients and caregivers. Home nurses are available not only to provide medical care but also to teach caregivers about tasks such as maintaining respirators, giving feedings, and moving patients to avoid painful skin problems and contractures. Home hospice nurses work in consultation with physicians to ensure proper medication, pain control, and other care affecting the quality of life of patients who wish to remain at home. The home hospice team can also counsel patients and caregivers about end-of-life issues.

Epidemiology

ALS is one of the most common neuromuscular diseases worldwide, and people of all races and ethnic backgrounds are affected. One or two out of 100,000 people develop ALS each year.[41] ALS most commonly strikes people between 40 and 60 years of age, but younger and older people can also develop the disease. Men are affected slightly more often than women.

Although the incidence of ALS is thought to be regionally uniform, there are three regions in the West Pacific where there has in the past been an elevated occurrence of ALS. This seems to be declining in recent decades. The largest is the area of Guam inhabited by the Chamorro people, who have historically had a high incidence (as much as 143 cases per 100,000 people per year) of a condition called Lytico-Bodig disease which is a combination of symptoms similar to ALS, parkinsonism, and dementia. Lytico-Bodig disease has been linked to the consumption of cycad seeds and in particular, the chemical found in cycad seeds, β-methylamino-L-alanine (BMAA).[42] Two more areas of increased incidence are West Papua and the Kii Peninsula of Japan.[43] [44]

Although there have been reports of several "clusters" including three American football players from the San Francisco 49ers, more than fifty football players in Italy,[45] three football-playing friends in the south of England,[46] and reports of conjugal (husband and wife) cases in the south of France,[47] [48] [49] [50] [51] these are statistically plausible chance events. Although many authors consider ALS to be caused by a combination of genetic and environmental risk factors, so far the latter have not been firmly identified, other than a higher risk with increasing age.

Etymology

Amyotrophic comes from the Greek language: *A-* means "no", *myo* refers to "muscle", and *trophic* means "nourishment"; *amyotrophic* therefore means "no muscle nourishment," which describes the characteristic atrophication of the sufferer's disused muscle tissue. *Lateral* identifies the areas in a person's spinal cord where portions of the nerve cells that are affected are located. As this area degenerates it leads to scarring or hardening ("sclerosis") in the region.

History

Timeline

Year	Event
1824	Charles Bell writes a report about ALS.[52]
1850	English scientist Augustus Waller describes the appearance of shriveled nerve fibers
1869	French doctor Jean-Martin Charcot first describes ALS in scientific literature[53]
1881	"Amyotrophic Lateral Sclerosis" is translated into English and published in a three-volume edition of Lectures on the Diseases of the Nervous System
1939	ALS becomes a *cause célèbre* in the United States when baseball legend Lou Gehrig's career—and, two years later, his life—is ended by the disease. He gives his farewell speech on 4 July 1939.[54]
1950s	ALS epidemic occurs among the Chamorro people on Guam
1991	Researchers link chromosome 21 to FALS (Familial ALS)
1993	SOD1 gene on chromosome 21 found to play a role in some cases of FALS
1996	Rilutek becomes the first FDA-approved drug for ALS
1998	The El Escorial criteria is developed as the standard for classifying ALS patient in clinical research
1999	The revised ALS Functional Rating Scale (ALSFRS-R) is published and soon becomes a gold standard measure for rating decline in ALS patient in clinical research
2011	Noncoding repeat expansions in C9ORF72 are found to be a major cause of ALS and frontotemporal dementia

Clinical research

A number of clinical trials are underway globally for ALS; a comprehensive listing of trials in the US can be found at ClinicalTrials.gov.

Thalidomide and Lenalidomide have shown efficacy in protecting motor neurons in transgenic (G93A) mice.[55]

KNS-760704 (Dexpramipexole) is under clinical investigation in ALS patients. It is hoped that the drug will have a neuroprotective effect. It is one enantiomer of pramipexole, which is approved for the treatment of Parkinson's disease and restless legs syndrome.[56] The single-enantiomer preparation is essentially inactive at dopamine receptors, is not dose limited by the potent dopaminergic properties of pramipexole.[57] Results of a Phase II clinical trial conducted by Knopp Neurosciences and involving 102 patients were reported in 2010; the trial found a dose-dependent slowing in loss of function.[58] A larger phase II trial conducted by Biogen found the drug to be safe, well tolerated, and associated with a dose-dependent slowing in the decline of ALS.[59] In January 2013, Biogen Idec announced that it was discontinuing its development of dexpramipexole in ALS due to lack of efficacy in a Phase III study.

A Phase II trial on talampanel was completed by Teva Pharmaceutical Industries in April 2010 however it was found to be negative for treatment viability.[60]

See also

- ALS Association
- ALS Society of Canada
- ALS Therapy Development Institute
- Motor Neurone Disease Association
- Muscular Dystrophy Association

References

[1] Dugdale DC, Hoch DB, Zieve D (August 27, 2010). "Amyotrophic lateral sclerosis" (http://www.ncbi.nlm.nih.gov/pubmedhealth/PMH0001708/). *A.D.A.M. Medical Encyclopedia.* .

[2] Phukan J, Pender NP, Hardiman O (2007). "Cognitive impairment in amyotrophic lateral sclerosis" (http://linkinghub.elsevier.com/retrieve/pii/S1474-4422(07)70265-X). *Lancet Neurol* **6** (11): 994–1003. doi:10.1016/S1474-4422(07)70265-X. PMID 17945153. .

[3] Error: Bad DOI specified!

[4] Error: Bad DOI specified!

[5] Turner MR, Parton MJ, Shaw CE, Leigh PN, Al-Chalabi A (2003). "Prolonged survival in motor neuron disease: a descriptive study of the King's database 1990–2002.". *J Neurol Neurosurg Psychiatry* **74**: 995–997.

[6] "Stephen Hawking serves as role model for ALS patients" (http://articles.cnn.com/2009-04-20/health/hawking.als_1_als-association-lou-gehrig-s-disease-motor-neuron-disease?_s=PM:HEALTH). CNN. 2009-04-20. .

[7] Sutedja NA, Fischer K, Veldink JH, van der Heijden GJ, Kromhout H, Heederik D, et al. (2009). "What we truly know about occupation as a risk factor for ALS: a critical and systematic review.". *Amyotrophic Lateral Sclerosis* **10**: 295–301.

[8] "Crucial Link Between Prions And ALS Discovered - May Transform Treatment" (http://www.medicalnewstoday.com/articles/234813.php). Medical News Today. 22 Sep 2011. . Retrieved 21 December 2012.

[9] Dejesus-Hernandez, M., et al., (2011). "Expanded GGGGCC Hexanucleotide Repeat in Noncoding Region of C9ORF72 Causes Chromosome 9p-Linked FTD and ALS.". *Neuron* **72** (2): 245–56.

[10] Majounie E., et al., (2012). "Frequency of the C9orf72 hexanucleotide repeat expansion in patients with amyotrophic lateral sclerosis and frontotemporal dementia: a cross-sectional study.". *Lancet Neurology* **11** (4): 323–330.

[11] Conwit, Robin A. (December 2006). "Preventing familial ALS: A clinical trial may be feasible but is an efficacy trial warranted?". *Journal of the Neurological Sciences* **251** (1–2): 1–2. doi:10.1016/j.jns.2006.07.009. ISSN 0022-510X. PMID 17070848.

[12] Al-Chalabi, Ammar; P. Nigel Leigh (August 2000). "Recent advances in amyotrophic lateral sclerosis". *Current Opinion in Neurology* **13** (4): 397–405. doi:10.1097/00019052-200008000-00006. ISSN 1473-6551. PMID 10970056.

[13] Battistini S, Ricci C, Lotti EM, Benigni M, Gagliardi S, Zucco R, Bondavalli M, Marcello N, Ceroni M, Cereda C (June 2010). "Severe familial ALS with a novel exon 4 mutation (L106F) in the SOD1 gene". *Journal of the Neurological Sciences* **293** (1): 112–115. doi:10.1016/j.jns.2010.03.009. PMID 20385392.

[14] Anderson P.M., et al., (1996). "Autosomal recessive adult-onset amyotrophic lateral sclerosis associated with homozygosity for Asp90Ala CuZn-superoxide dismutase mutation, A clinical and genealogical study of 36 patients.". *Brain* **119**: 1153–1172.

[15] Error: Bad DOI specified!

[16] Error: Bad DOI specified!

[17] Error: Bad DOI specified!

[18] Error: Bad DOI specified!

[19] Deng, HX; Chen, W, Hong, ST, Boycott, KM, Gorrie, GH, Siddique, N, Yang, Y, Fecto, F, Shi, Y, Zhai, H, Jiang, H, Hirano, M, Rampersaud, E, Jansen, GH, Donkervoort, S, Bigio, EH, Brooks, BR, Ajroud, K, Sufit, RL, Haines, JL, Mugnaini, E, Pericak-Vance, MA, Siddique, T (2011-08-21). "Mutations in UBQLN2 cause dominant X-linked juvenile and adult onset ALS and ALS/dementia". *Nature* **477** (7363): 211–5. doi:10.1038/nature10353. PMC 3169705. PMID 21857683.

[20] Reaume A, Elliott J, Hoffman E, Kowall N, Ferrante R, Siwek D, Wilcox H, Flood D, Beal M, Brown R, Scott R, Snider W (1996). "Motor neurons in Cu/Zn superoxide dismutase-deficient mice develop normally but exhibit enhanced cell death after axonal injury". *Nat Genet* **13** (1): 43–7. doi:10.1038/ng0596-43. PMID 8673102.

[21] Bruijn L, Houseweart M, Kato S, Anderson K, Anderson S, Ohama E, Reaume A, Scott R, Cleveland D (1998). "Aggregation and motor neuron toxicity of an ALS-linked SOD1 mutant independent from wild-type SOD1". *Science* **281** (5384): 1851–4. doi:10.1126/science.281.5384.1851. PMID 9743498.

[22] Furukawa Y, Fu R, Deng H, Siddique T, O'Halloran T (2006). "Disulfide cross-linked protein represents a significant fraction of ALS-associated Cu, Zn-superoxide dismutase aggregates in spinal cords of model mice". *Proc Natl Acad Sci USA* **103** (18): 7148–53. doi:10.1073/pnas.0602048103. PMC 1447524. PMID 16636274.

[23] Boillée S, Vande Velde C, Cleveland D (2006). "ALS: a disease of motor neurons and their nonneuronal neighbors". *Neuron* **52** (1): 39–59. doi:10.1016/j.neuron.2006.09.018. PMID 17015226.

[24] Hansel Y, Ackerl M, Stanek G. (1995). "ALS-like sequelae in chronic neuroborreliosis". *Wien Med Wochenschr.* **145** (7–8): 186–8. PMID 7610670.

[25] el Alaoui-Faris M, Medejel A, al Zemmouri K, Yahyaoui M, Chkili T (1990). "Amyotrophic lateral sclerosis syndrome of syphilitic origin. 5 cases". *Rev Neurol (Paris)* **146** (1): 41–4. PMID 2408129.

[26] Umanekii KG, Dekonenko EP (1983). "Structure of progressive forms of tick-borne encephalitis". *Zh Nevropatol Psikhiatr Im S S Korsakova.* **83** (8): 1173–9. PMID 6414202.

[27] Silani, V.; Messina, S.; Poletti, B.; Morelli, C.; Doretti, A.; Ticozzi, N.; Maderna, L. (2011). "The diagnosis of Amyotrophic lateral sclerosis in 2010". *Archives italiennes de biologie* **149** (1): 5–27. doi:10.4449/aib.v149i1.1260. PMID 21412713.

[28] Eisen, A. (2002). "Amyotrophic lateral sclerosis: A review" (http://www.bcmj.org/article/amyotrophic-lateral-sclerosis-review). *BCMJ* **44** (7): 362–366. .

[29] Error: Bad DOI specified!

[30] Error: Bad DOI specified!

[31] Al-Asmi, A.; Nandhagopal, R.; Jacob, P. C.; Gujjar, A. (2012). "Misdiagnosis of Myasthenia Gravis and Subsequent Clinical Implication: A case report and review of literature". *Sultan Qaboos University medical journal* **12** (1): 103–108. PMC 3286704. PMID 22375266.

[32] http://misc.medscape.com/pi/android/medscapeapp/html/A1170810-business.html

[33] http://www.lems.com/what_is_lems

[34] Carlesi, C; Pasquali, L, Piazza, S, Lo Gerfo, A, Caldarazzo Ienco, E, Alessi, R, Fornai, F, Siciliano, G (March 2011). "Strategies for clinical approach to neurodegeneration in Amyotrophic lateral sclerosis". *Archives italiennes de biologie* **149** (1): 151–67. doi:10.4449/aib.v149i1.1267. PMID 21412722.

[35] Miller, RG; Mitchell JD, Lyon M, Moore DH, G (2007). Miller, Robert G. ed. "Riluzole for amyotrophic lateral sclerosis (ALS)/motor neuron disease (MND)". *Cochrane Database of Systematic Reviews* (1): CD001447. doi:10.1002/14651858.CD001447.pub2. PMID 17253460.

[36] Lewis, M. & Rushanan, S. (2007). "The role of physical therapy and occupational therapy in the treatment of Amyotrophic Lateral Sclerosis". *NeuroRehabilitation* **22** (6): 451–461. PMID 18198431.

[37] Kasarskis EJ, Berryman S, Vanderleest JG, Schneider AR, McClain CJ (Jan 1996). "Nutritional status of patients with amyotrophic lateral sclerosis: relation to the proximity of death" (http://www.ajcn.org/cgi/pmidlookup?view=long&pmid=8604660). *Am J Clin Nutr.* **63** (1): 130–7. PMID 8604660. .

[38] Hamadeh MJ, Rodriguez MC, Kaczor JJ, Tarnopolsky MA (Feb 2005). "Caloric restriction transiently improves motor performance but hastens clinical onset of disease in the Cu/Zn-superoxide dismutase mutant G93A mouse". *Muscle Nerve* **31** (2): 214–20. doi:10.1002/mus.20255. PMID 15625688.

[39] Slowie LA, Paige MS, Antel JP (Jul 1983). "Nutritional considerations in the management of patients with amyotrophic lateral sclerosis (ALS)". *J Am Diet Assoc* **83** (1): 44–7. PMID 6863783.

[40] Sviri S, Linton DM, Van Heerden PV (Jun 2005). "Non-invasive Mechanical Ventilation Enhances Patient Autonomy in Decision-Making Regarding Chronic Ventilation". *Critical Care and Resuscitation* **7** (2): 116–118. PMID 16548804.

[41] "ALS Topic Overview" (http://www.webmd.com/brain/tc/Amyotrophic-Lateral-Sclerosis-ALS-Topic-Overview). Archived (http://web.archive.org/web/20080501194730/http://www.webmd.com/brain/tc/amyotrophic-lateral-sclerosis-als-topic-overview) from the original on 1 May 2008. . Retrieved 2008-05-01.

[42] Reed D, Labarthe D, Chen KM, Stallones R (Jan 1987). "A cohort study of amyotrophic lateral sclerosis and parkinsonism-dementia on Guam and Rota" (http://aje.oxfordjournals.org/cgi/pmidlookup?view=long&pmid=3788958). *Am J Epidemiol.* **125** (1): 92–100. PMID 3788958. .

[43] S. Kuzuhara, Y. Kokubo P3-146Marked increase of parkinsonism-dementia (P-D) phenotypes in the high incidence amyotrophic lateral sclerosis (ALS) focus in the Kii peninsula of Japan. Alzheimer's and Dementia, Volume 2, Issue 3, Pages S417-S417

[44] Spencer PS, Palmer VS, Ludolph AC (Aug 2005). "On the decline and etiology of high-incidence motor system disease in West Papua (southwest New Guinea)". *Mov. Disord.* **20** (Suppl 12): S119–26. doi:10.1002/mds.20552. PMID 16092101.

[45] "Sla, indagini nei club. Pesticidi nel mirino" (http://www.corriere.it/sport/08_ottobre_03/sla_indagine_pesticidi_fd04f986-911c-11dd-9f28-00144f02aabc.shtml). Archived (http://web.archive.org/web/20081003220654/http://www.corriere.it/sport/08_ottobre_03/sla_indagine_pesticidi_fd04f986-911c-11dd-9f28-00144f02aabc.shtml) from the original on 3 October 2008. . Retrieved 2008-10-02.

[46] Wicks P, Abrahams S, Masi D, Hejda-Forde S, Leigh PN & Goldstein LH (2005) The Prevalence of Depression and Anxiety in MND, Amyotrophic Lateral Sclerosis and other Motor Neuron Disorders, Volume 6, Supplement 1, p. 147

[47] Rachele MG, Mascia V, Tacconi P, Dessi N, Marrosu F (April 1998). "Conjugal amyotrophic lateral sclerosis: a report on a couple from Sardinia, Italy". *Ital J Neurol Sci.* **19** (2): 97–100. doi:10.1007/BF02427565. PMID 10935845.

[48] Poloni M, Micheli A, Facchetti D, Mai R, Ceriani F (April 1997). "Conjugal amyotrophic lateral sclerosis: toxic clustering or change?". *Ital J Neurol Sci.* **18** (2): 109–12. doi:10.1007/BF01999572. PMID 9239532.

[49] Camu W, Cadilhac J, Billiard M. (March 1994). "Conjugal amyotrophic lateral sclerosis: a report on two couples from southern France". *Neurology* **44** (3 Pt 1): 547–8. PMID 8145930.

[50] Cornblath DR, Kurland LT, Boylan KB, Morrison L, Radhakrishnan K, Montgomery M. (November 1993). "Conjugal amyotrophic lateral sclerosis: report of a young married couple". *Neurology* **43** (11): 2378–80. PMID 8232960.

[51] Corcia P, Jafari-Schluep HF, Lardillier D, Mazyad H, Giraud P, Clavelou P, Pouget J, Camu W (November 2003). "A clustering of conjugal amyotrophic lateral sclerosis in southeastern France". *Neurol.* **60** (4): 553–7. doi:10.1001/archneur.60.4.553. PMID 12707069.

[52] Tyler HR, Shefner J. Amyotrophic lateral sclerosis. Handb Clin Neurol. 1991;15:169–215. Serial publication.

[53] Rowland LP (March 2001). "How amyotrophic lateral sclerosis got its name: the clinical-pathologic genius of Jean-Martin Charcot" (http://archneur.ama-assn.org/cgi/content/extract/58/3/512). *Arch. Neurol.* **58** (3): 512–5. doi:10.1001/archneur.58.3.512. PMID 11255459. .

[54] "Farewell Speech" (http://www.lougehrig.com/about/speech.htm). lougehrig.com. 4 July 1939. Archived (http://web.archive.org/web/20080412123358/http://www.lougehrig.com/about/speech.htm) from the original on 12 April 2008. . Retrieved 16 April 2008.

[55] *The Journal of Neuroscience* **26** (9): 2467-2473. March 1 2006. http://www.jneurosci.org/content/26/9/2467.full.pdf+html.

[56] Abramova NA et al. (2002 Feb 15). "Inhibition by R(+) or S(-) pramipexole of caspase activation and cell death induced by methylpyridinium ion or beta amyloid peptide in SH-SY5Y neuroblastoma". *J Neurosci Res* **67** (4): 494–500. PMID 11835316.

[57] Error: Bad DOI specified!

[58] Error: Bad DOI specified!

[59] Error: Bad DOI specified!

[60] "Talampanel for Amyotrophic Lateral Sclerosis (ALS)". ClinicalTrials.gov.

Further reading

- "ALS Hope Foundation" (http://www.alshopefoundation.org/). Archived (http://web.archive.org/web/20080512012521/http://www.alshopefoundation.org/) from the original on 12 May 2008. Retrieved 2008-06-21. "Dedicated to the care and cure of people with Lou Gehrig's Disease. (from site page us.php)"
- "Lou Gehrig: The Official Web Site" (http://www.lougehrig.com). CMG Worldwide. Archived (http://web.archive.org/web/20080509101328/http://www.lougehrig.com/) from the original on 9 May 2008. Retrieved 2008-06-21. "The Official Web site of Lou Gehrig is an informational Web site intended to honor the life, the legend and the career of Lou Gehrig. (from site page siteinfo/index.htm)"
- Patrick Aebischer; Ann C. Kato (November 2007). "Playing defense against Lou Gehrig's Disease" (http://www.sciam.com/article.cfm?id=playing-defense-against-l) (Paper). *Scientific American* (Verlagsgruppe Georg von Holtzbrinck): pp. 86–93. Retrieved 2008-06-21. "Researchers have proposed potential therapies for a paralyzing disorder once thought to be untreatable (sub-title)"

External links

- Medline Plus article on ALS (https://www.nlm.nih.gov/medlineplus/amyotrophiclateralsclerosis.html)

Article Sources and Contributors

Recessive *Source*: http://en.wikipedia.org/w/index.php?title=Recessive *Contributors*: Adrian J. Hunter, Brunodiaz79, ChocolateBall, Christian75, CityOfSilver, Dr d12, Facts707, FilipeS, Gaius Cornelius, Gurch, Gwickwire, Heron, Impyrean, Kalaiarasy, Kashmiri, Kevin Dorner, LuK3, Madeleine Price Ball, Medeis, Michaelzeng7, Morwen, Nuarbat, Ohiostandard, Openmouth, RandomAct, Redirect fixer, Shakiestone, The Illusive Man, Weedwhacker128, Y12J, 49 anonymous edits

Spinal muscular atrophy *Source*: http://en.wikipedia.org/w/index.php?title=Spinal_muscular_atrophy *Contributors*: Andrew73, Arcadian, Bearflag70, Beccaviola, Bjornman, Calaka, Coinmanj, Daniel Mietchen, Escape Orbit, Henry A Stanley, Huatwin, Jennes83, Kashmiri, Kejood, Khazar, Kids Neuro Doc, Kjkolb, Littrans, Mikael Häggström, Naseem abi shaheen, Nbauman, Paul A, Pauli133, Rigadoun, Sisyphustkd, Sylwia Ufnalska, ToMMiTTo, דוד55, 25 anonymous edits

Survival motor neuron spinal muscular atrophy *Source*: http://en.wikipedia.org/w/index.php?title=Survival_motor_neuron_spinal_muscular_atrophy *Contributors*: Andrew73, Arcadian, Bearflag70, Beccaviola, Bjornman, Calaka, Coinmanj, Daniel Mietchen, Escape Orbit, Henry A Stanley, Huatwin, Jennes83, Kashmiri, Kejood, Khazar, Kids Neuro Doc, Kjkolb, Littrans, Mikael Häggström, Naseem abi shaheen, Nbauman, Paul A, Pauli133, Rigadoun, Sisyphustkd, Sylwia Ufnalska, ToMMiTTo, דוד55, 25 anonymous edits

Motor neurone disease *Source*: http://en.wikipedia.org/w/index.php?title=Motor_neurone_disease *Contributors*: 144Bob, 1exec1, 2112 rush, A phone with appeal!, A876, AHands, ALAUK, Aaronwinborn, Abarry, Adamahill, Adrealtor, Aervanath, Against the current, Airplaneman, Aj911, Alansohn, Alecabio497, Alex Bakharev, Aliiisha, Alpha Quadrant (alt), Alstdf, Amesville, Amire80, Andrew73, Antandrus, Antarctic-adventurer, Anthony Appleyard, Anthonyhcole, Aok82, ApersOn, Arcadian, Are1981, Art8641, Aruton, Ashbury305, Avanze, Aytrus, B, B.d.mills, BD2412, BG56789, Bagatelle, Barek, Barwick Joans, Bdesham, BelsKr, Bebestooge44, Ben.Spaetzel, Bender235, Bennybp, Berean Hunter, Between My Ken, Beveleig, BiT, Blanchardb, Bmf 51, Bobblewik, Bobo192, Bork, Brainhell, Braum, Brian1979, Bstandley, Btharper1221, Burnwelk, Busiken, CDN99, Cadsuane Melaidhrin, CalendarWatcher, CaliforniaLyme, Calmer Waters, Calton, CambridgeBayWeather, Camden7, Can't sleep, clown will eat me, Carolfrog, Casper2k3, Cat-five, Catgut, Celestra, Ceyockey, Chachilongbow, Chao, Cheryl Mason, Chickennugget1234567890000, Chris 73, Chris Capoccia, Chris the speller, Christidy, Circumspect, Cjman546, Ckaiserca, Ckim2, Cole.jeff, Colin, Colinportnuff, Commalz, CompassionateCareALS, Craig Pemberton, Crazynanny, Cureden, Cwcollier, DARTH SIDIOUS 2, DBigXray, DVdm, Dale Arnett, DanAtNR, Danste182, Dawgsplayinpoka, Daysleeper47, Delirium, Delldot, Dgonzales138, Dingno, Discospinster, Distantsuns, Diza, Dl2000, DocJohnny, DoctorEric, Doctorindy, Dominus, Doug4422, Dougofborg, Dr Dextrous, Dr Geurnice, Dr. Interesting, Dr.Milánkovits, Dreadstar, Drewigg, Drsamir, Dudesleeper, Dwimble1, Dylan38, Dynaflow, Eastfrisian, Ebyabe, Eddy23, EdwardsQueensPT2013, El monty, EmetHodge, Empyre720, Engkjt, Enigmaman, Epbr123, Eric.laporta, EricaValtory, Esperant, Esrever, Etaicq, Ethanwarshow, Faigl.ladislav, Fenwickswimmer, Fetchcomms, Fetor Beltez, Fifid, Fifth Rider, Finduilas 09, Fingerz, Flavienck, Floaterfluss, Floydspinky71, Fminow, Fordmadoxfraud, Fourthy, Foxhound66, Frank, Free smyrnan, Freewol, Froid, Furrykef, Fxmastermind, Gadfium, Garion96, Gbutler77, Gcgmd, GeeJo, Geo12a, Georgethe23rd, Gfmer, Giftlite, Gigano, Gigemag76, GinaDana, Gio69, Gjensendk, GoShow, Gobonobo, Great Scott, Greensburger, GregorB, Gtadoc, Guffydrawers, Gunitkaratemasta, Gurch, Gus Tuck, Guðsþegn, Gyre, Haikaa, Hateless, Hawesinsky, Headbomb, Hede2000, HelenKMarks, Heracles31, Hillsbro, Hirschn, HistoryMan22, HopeCenterWustl, Hu12, Hydrargyrum, Ian Goddard, Icairns, Iced Kola, Ilaiho, Ildkugle, Illia Connell, Indian1970, Iolathe, J-boogie, J.delanoy, JHUbme24, JSpung, JWSchmidt, JaGa, James pic, Jamoche, Jamorel, Jbaylor, Jeff Muscato, Jeff Silvers, Jeff3000, Jeffgh88, Jeriaska, Jeromeleonard, Jfdwolff, Jim1138, JimmyOrangeSeed, Jlawilliams, Jmh649, JoanneB, Joefromrandb, John Rendor, John Vandenberg, John of Reading, JohnJHenderson, Jonathansamuel, Jonpro, Jooler, Jpatokal, Julesd, Juliancolton, Jumbolino, Junocola, JustJuthan, Justin Eiler, Jytdog, K4948, Kaimiddleton, Karyyk, Kashmiri, Kasper2006, Katalaveno, Kate Carter, Katydidit, Ke4roh, Keenan Pepper, Kerowyn, Khvalamde, Kidlittle, Kimberstrike, Kingfish, Kirkrules, Kitch, Kjkolb, Knowledgeum, Koavf, Kslays, Kuang Eleven, Kummi, Kvn8907, LOL, LaFoiblesse, Lacertuslecti, Lambiam, Lapisphil, Lary Walker, LeadSongDog, LedgendGamer, Leejabramson, Leon7, Leujohn, Lientje111, Light current, Liisamackey, LilHelpa, LindsayH, Livingat45north, Lizzieb904, Looie496, Lord Hawk, Lostlogicx, Lproven, Lshanahan, Lugnuts, Luqui, Luvkush4210, Luxomni, M0s6p, MER-C, MKoltnow, MMX, Madhero88, Magioladitis, Makelelecba, Mamatz, Manushand, Markmc, Markthemac, Marskuzz, Martarius, MartinezMD, MarxistRevolutionary, Mashford, Masparasol, Mastergurosp, Matthew Chi Lee, MatthewMain, Mattweng, Mauricev, Mazca, Megadude45, Mekeretrig, Melaen, Mermaid from the Baltic Sea, Merrymairi, Meta09, Mgiganteus1, Michael Daly, Mike.lifeguard, Mild Bill Hiccup, Mintguy, Mjp202, Mkamensek, Mnkyho92, Moe Epsilon, Monkey features, Moreschi, Mr.Z-man, Mrvaughan, MusiCitizen, Musicmansuperman, Mwalcoff, Mz, Möchtegern, Nagelfar, NawlinWiki, Nbarth, Nelly Furtado, Netkinetic, Neutrall, New World Man, Nickyus, Nightscream, Nightsky, Nihiltres, Nilloc, Nina, Nishkid64, Nivix, Noah Salzman, Nodar95, NotWith, Npnunda, Nyttend, OJSlaughter, Oanjao, Ocatecir, OccamzRazor, OhanaUnited, Ojii-san, Omnipotent person, Orphan Wiki, Orphu of io, Otvaltak, Oxymoron83, Patrickbowman, PaulWicks, Peacedance, Pekingduck888, Peter Greenwell, Pfistermeister, Ph.eyes, PhilKnight, Philip Trueman, Phorbol, Phoénix, Pigman, Polycarp, Posidonious, Postlewaight, Postmodern Beatnik, Postoak, Poule, Prashanthns, PrestonH, Prezbo, Princesschickencat, Puchiko, Puffin, Qdiderot, QuiteUnusual, Qxz, RA0808, RDBrown, RG2, Radamanthe81, Raggaga, Raja99, Randall222, RandomP, Rangek, RaspberryKlonopin, Ratinator939, Raulthepoolboy, Ravedave, Raymax, Renamed vandal 85, RexNL, ReyBrujo, Rich Farmbrough, Richar4034, Richardcavell, Richardjames444, Richwales, Riley Huntley, Rjwilmsi, Rm1271, Robinatron, Robmelone, Rod57, RoyBatty42, Rreagan007, Ruthiedee, S, Salmar, Sam Blacketer, Samantha1961, Samir, SandyGeorgia, Sanjpatel1, Sannse, Sasata, Save tha sasquatchas, Sbrools, Sean.hoyland, SeanMack, Seans Potato Business, Ser Amantio di Nicolao, Sfdavide, Sgtmacdonald102079, Shambalala, Shocking Blue, Sidcool1234, Siennadog, Sintaku, Sirnoze, Skamecrazy123, Skinsmoke, Slashme, Slawojarek, Slp1, Snowmanradio, Soames, Someguy1221, Sonjaaa, Spariant, Sparntez, SpiderJon, Srgregson, Stemonitis, StephenBuxton, Stevechimo, Steven Zhang, Stoiko Stoilov, Strongbadmanofme, Sunshynesupaman, Syrthiss, T-borg, THEGR814EVER, Takamine45, Teeninvestor, Teh newbie, Temporaluser, TenOfAllTrades, Tgeairn, The High Fin Sperm Whale, The Thing That Should Not Be, TheHYPO, Theflyer, Thief12, Thingg, Thisglad, Thomas Larsen, Thumperward, Timwi, Tinabtw, Tiptoety, Tony1, Trusilver, TrustTruth, Tukkeramn, Tumblingsky, Turtlemouth, Twas Now, Ucucha, Ulape, Uploadvirus, Velella, Velho, Velocipedia, Versageek, Viper h, Viridian, Vmulligan, VolatileChemical, Vrenator, W guice, WMarsh, Wannabe13, Wavelength, Wayward, Wdfarmer, Wfbyankee, Whatamldoing, Whpq, Wiki alf, Wiki emma johnson, WikiPier, Wikieditorforversailles, Wikiman208, Wikipelli, WilliamJE, Wilsongirl00, Wimt, Winhunter, Wisdom89, WolfmanSF, Woohookitty, Word31, WorldWide Update, Wouterstomp, Wutime, Yamamoto 15, Yandman, Yannako, Yobol, Yornanelat, Ysangkok, Zawersh, Zigzag1, Zzyzx11, דוד55, علی ویی، امنی،
1305 anonymous edits

Motor neurone disease *Source*: http://en.wikipedia.org/w/index.php?title=Motor_neurone_disease *Contributors*: 144Bob, 1exec1, 2112 rush, A phone with appeal!, A876, AHands, ALAUK, Aaronwinborn, Abarry, Adamahill, Adrealtor, Aervanath, Against the current, Airplaneman, Aj911, Alansohn, Alecabio497, Alex Bakharev, Aliiisha, Alpha Quadrant (alt), Alstdf, Amesville, Amire80, Andrew73, Antandrus, Antarctic-adventurer, Anthony Appleyard, Anthonyhcole, Aok82, ApersOn, Arcadian, Are1981, Art8641, Aruton, Ashbury305, Avanze, Aytrus, B, B.d.mills, BD2412, BG56789, Bagatelle, Barek, Barwick Joans, Bdesham, BelsKr, Bebestooge44, Ben.Spaetzel, Bender235, Bennybp, Berean Hunter, Between My Ken, Beveleig, BiT, Blanchardb, Bmf 51, Bobblewik, Bobo192, Bork, Brainhell, Braum, Brian1979, Bstandley, Btharper1221, Burnwelk, Busiken, CDN99, Cadsuane Melaidhrin, CalendarWatcher, CaliforniaLyme, Calmer Waters, Calton, CambridgeBayWeather, Camden7, Can't sleep, clown will eat me, Carolfrog, Casper2k3, Cat-five, Catgut, Celestra, Ceyockey, Chachilongbow, Chao, Cheryl Mason, Chickennugget1234567890000, Chris 73, Chris Capoccia, Chris the speller, Christidy, Circumspect, Cjman546, Ckaiserca, Ckim2, Cole.jeff, Colin, Colinportnuff, Commalz, CompassionateCareALS, Craig Pemberton, Crazynanny, Cureden, Cwcollier, DARTH SIDIOUS 2, DBigXray, DVdm, Dale Arnett, DanAtNR, Danste182, Dawgsplayinpoka, Daysleeper47, Delirium, Delldot, Dgonzales138, Dingno, Discospinster, Distantsuns, Diza, Dl2000, DocJohnny, DoctorEric, Doctorindy, Dominus, Doug4422, Dougofborg, Dr Dextrous, Dr Geurnice, Dr. Interesting, Dr.Milánkovits, Dreadstar, Drewigg, Drsamir, Dudesleeper, Dwimble1, Dylan38, Dynaflow, Eastfrisian, Ebyabe, Eddy23, EdwardsQueensPT2013, El monty, EmetHodge, Empyre720, Engkjt, Enigmaman, Epbr123, Eric.laporta, EricaValtory, Esperant, Esrever, Etaicq, Ethanwarshow, Faigl.ladislav, Fenwickswimmer, Fetchcomms, Fetor Beltez, Fifid, Fifth Rider, Finduilas 09, Fingerz, Flavienck, Floaterfluss, Floydspinky71, Fminow, Fordmadoxfraud, Fourthy, Foxhound66, Frank, Free smyrnan, Freewol, Froid, Furrykef, Fxmastermind, Gadfium, Garion96, Gbutler77, Gcgmd, GeeJo, Geo12a, Georgethe23rd, Gfmer, Giftlite, Gigano, Gigemag76, GinaDana, Gio69, Gjensendk, GoShow, Gobonobo, Great Scott, Greensburger, GregorB, Gtadoc, Guffydrawers, Gunitkaratemasta, Gurch, Gus Tuck, Guðsþegn, Gyre, Haikaa, Hateless, Hawesinsky, Headbomb, Hede2000, HelenKMarks, Heracles31, Hillsbro, Hirschn, HistoryMan22, HopeCenterWustl, Hu12, Hydrargyrum, Ian Goddard, Icairns, Iced Kola, Ilaiho, Ildkugle, Illia Connell, Indian1970, Iolathe, J-boogie, J.delanoy, JHUbme24, JSpung, JWSchmidt, JaGa, James pic, Jamoche, Jamorel, Jbaylor, Jeff Muscato, Jeff Silvers, Jeff3000, Jeffgh88, Jeriaska, Jeromeleonard, Jfdwolff, Jim1138, JimmyOrangeSeed, Jlawilliams, Jmh649, JoanneB, Joefromrandb, John Rendor, John Vandenberg, John of Reading, JohnJHenderson, Jonathansamuel, Jonpro, Jooler, Jpatokal, Julesd, Juliancolton, Jumbolino, Junocola, JustJuthan, Justin Eiler, Jytdog, K4948, Kaimiddleton, Karyyk, Kashmiri, Kasper2006, Katalaveno, Kate Carter, Katydidit, Ke4roh, Keenan Pepper, Kerowyn, Khvalamde, Kidlittle, Kimberstrike, Kingfish, Kirkrules, Kitch, Kjkolb, Knowledgeum, Koavf, Kslays, Kuang Eleven, Kummi, Kvn8907, LOL, LaFoiblesse, Lacertuslecti, Lambiam, Lapisphil, Lary Walker, LeadSongDog, LedgendGamer, Leejabramson, Leon7, Leujohn, Lientje111, Light current, Liisamackey, LilHelpa, LindsayH, Livingat45north, Lizzieb904, Looie496, Lord Hawk, Lostlogicx, Lproven, Lshanahan, Lugnuts, Luqui, Luvkush4210, Luxomni, M0s6p, MER-C, MKoltnow, MMX, Madhero88, Magioladitis, Makelelecba, Mamatz, Manushand, Markmc, Markthemac, Marskuzz, Martarius, MartinezMD, MarxistRevolutionary, Mashford, Masparasol, Mastergurosp, Matthew Chi Lee, MatthewMain, Mattweng, Mauricev, Mazca, Megadude45, Mekeretrig, Melaen, Mermaid from the Baltic Sea, Merrymairi, Meta09, Mgiganteus1, Michael Daly, Mike.lifeguard, Mild Bill Hiccup, Mintguy, Mjp202, Mkamensek, Mnkyho92, Moe Epsilon, Monkey features, Moreschi, Mr.Z-man, Mrvaughan, MusiCitizen, Musicmansuperman, Mwalcoff, Mz, Möchtegern, Nagelfar, NawlinWiki, Nbarth, Nelly Furtado, Netkinetic, Neutrall, New World Man, Nickyus, Nightscream, Nightsky, Nihiltres, Nilloc, Nina, Nishkid64, Nivix, Noah Salzman, Nodar95, NotWith, Npnunda, Nyttend, OJSlaughter, Oanjao, Ocatecir, OccamzRazor, OhanaUnited, Ojii-san, Omnipotent person, Orphan Wiki, Orphu of io, Otvaltak, Oxymoron83, Patrickbowman, PaulWicks, Peacedance, Pekingduck888, Peter Greenwell, Pfistermeister, Ph.eyes, PhilKnight, Philip Trueman, Phorbol, Phoénix, Pigman, Polycarp, Posidonious, Postlewaight, Postmodern Beatnik, Postoak, Poule, Prashanthns, PrestonH, Prezbo, Princesschickencat, Puchiko, Puffin, Qdiderot, QuiteUnusual, Qxz, RA0808, RDBrown, RG2, Radamanthe81, Raggaga, Raja99, Randall222, RandomP, Rangek, RaspberryKlonopin, Ratinator939, Raulthepoolboy, Ravedave, Raymax, Renamed vandal 85, RexNL, ReyBrujo, Rich Farmbrough, Richar4034, Richardcavell, Richardjames444, Richwales, Riley Huntley, Rjwilmsi, Rm1271, Robinatron, Robmelone, Rod57, RoyBatty42, Rreagan007, Ruthiedee, S, Salmar, Sam Blacketer, Samantha1961, Samir, SandyGeorgia, Sanjpatel1, Sannse, Sasata, Save tha sasquatchas, Sbrools, Sean.hoyland, SeanMack, Seans Potato Business, Ser Amantio di Nicolao, Sfdavide, Sgtmacdonald102079, Shambalala, Shocking Blue, Sidcool1234, Siennadog, Sintaku, Sirnoze, Skamecrazy123, Skinsmoke, Slashme, Slawojarek, Slp1, Snowmanradio, Soames, Someguy1221, Sonjaaa, Spariant, Sparntez, SpiderJon, Srgregson, Stemonitis, StephenBuxton, Stevechimo, Steven Zhang, Stoiko Stoilov, Strongbadmanofme, Sunshynesupaman, Syrthiss, T-borg, THEGR814EVER, Takamine45, Teeninvestor, Teh newbie, Temporaluser, TenOfAllTrades, Tgeairn, The High Fin Sperm Whale, The Thing That Should Not Be, TheHYPO, Theflyer, Thief12, Thingg, Thisglad, Thomas Larsen, Thumperward, Timwi, Tinabtw, Tiptoety, Tony1, Trusilver, TrustTruth, Tukkeramn, Tumblingsky, Turtlemouth, Twas Now, Ucucha, Ulape, Uploadvirus, Velella, Velho, Velocipedia, Versageek, Viper h, Viridian, Vmulligan, VolatileChemical, Vrenator, W guice, WMarsh, Wannabe13, Wavelength, Wayward, Wdfarmer, Wfbyankee,

WhatamIdoing, Whpq, Wiki alf, Wiki emma johnson, WikiPier, Wikieditorforversailles, Wikiman208, Wikipelli, WilliamJE, Wilsongirl00, Wimt, Winhunter, Wisdom89, WolfmanSF, Woohookitty, Word31, WorldWide Update, Wouterstomp, Wutime, Yamamoto 15, Yandman, Yannako, Yobol, Yornanelat, Ysangkok, Zawersh, Zigzag1, Zzyzx11, דוד55, علی ویی، مانی, 1305 anonymous edits

Image Sources, Licenses and Contributors

Image:Autorecessive.svg *Source*: http://en.wikipedia.org/w/index.php?title=File:Autorecessive.svg *License*: unknown *Contributors*: Bender235, Cburnett, CiaPan, Hystrix, Kilom691, LordT, The Evil IP address, Zlir'a, 8 anonymous edits

File:Polio spinal diagram.PNG *Source*: http://en.wikipedia.org/w/index.php?title=File:Polio_spinal_diagram.PNG *License*: unknown *Contributors*: User:DO11.10

Image:Autosomal recessive - en.svg *Source*: http://en.wikipedia.org/w/index.php?title=File:Autosomal_recessive_-_en.svg *License*: unknown *Contributors*: User:Domaina, User:Kashmiri

File:ALS Coronal.jpg *Source*: http://en.wikipedia.org/w/index.php?title=File:ALS_Coronal.jpg *License*: unknown *Contributors*: User:Frank Gaillard

File:ALS cross.jpg *Source*: http://en.wikipedia.org/w/index.php?title=File:ALS_cross.jpg *License*: unknown *Contributors*: User:Frank Gaillard

GNU Free Documentation License Version 1.2, November 2002 Copyright (C) 2000,2001,2002 Free Software Foundation, Inc. 59 Temple Place, Suite 330, Boston, MA 02111-1307 USA Everyone is permitted to copy and distribute verbatim copies of this license document, but changing it is not allowed.

0. PREAMBLE

The purpose of this License is to make a manual, textbook, or other functional and useful document "free" in the sense of freedom: to assure everyone the effective freedom to copy and redistribute it, with or without modifying it, either commercially or noncommercially. Secondarily, this License preserves for the author and publisher a way to get credit for their work, while not being considered responsible for modifications made by others. This License is a kind of "copyleft", which means that derivative works of the document must themselves be free in the same sense. It complements the GNU General Public License, which is a copyleft license designed for free software. We have designed this License in order to use it for manuals for free software, because free software needs free documentation: a free program should come with manuals providing the same freedoms that the software does. But this License is not limited to software manuals; it can be used for any textual work, regardless of subject matter or whether it is published as a printed book. We recommend this License principally for works whose purpose is instruction or reference.

1. APPLICABILITY AND DEFINITIONS

This License applies to any manual or other work, in any medium, that contains a notice placed by the copyright holder saying it can be distributed under the terms of this License. Such a notice grants a world-wide, royalty-free license, unlimited in duration, to use that work under the conditions stated herein. The "Document", below, refers to any such manual or work. Any member of the public is a licensee, and is addressed as "you". You accept the license if you copy, modify or distribute the work in a way requiring permission under copyright law. A "Modified Version" of the Document means any work containing the Document or a portion of it, either copied verbatim, or with modifications and/or translated into another language. A "Secondary Section" is a named appendix or a front-matter section of the Document that deals exclusively with the relationship of the publishers or authors of the Document to the Document's overall subject (or to related matters) and contains nothing that could fall directly within that overall subject. (Thus, if the Document is in part a textbook of mathematics, a Secondary Section may not explain any mathematics.) The relationship could be a matter of historical connection with the subject or with related matters, or of legal, commercial, philosophical, ethical or political position regarding them. The "Invariant Sections" are certain Secondary Sections whose titles are designated, as being those of Invariant Sections, in the notice that says that the Document is released under this License. If a section does not fit the above definition of Secondary then it is not allowed to be designated as Invariant. The Document may contain zero Invariant Sections. If the Document does not identify any Invariant Sections then there are none. The "Cover Texts" are certain short passages of text that are listed, as Front-Cover Texts or Back-Cover Texts, in the notice that says that the Document is released under this License. A Front-Cover Text may be at most 5 words, and a Back-Cover Text may be at most 25 words. A "Transparent" copy of the Document means a machine-readable copy, represented in a format whose specification is available to the general public, that is suitable for revising the document straightforwardly with generic text editors or (for images composed of pixels) generic paint programs or (for drawings) some widely available drawing editor, and that is suitable for input to text formatters or for automatic translation to a variety of formats suitable for input to text formatters. A copy made in an otherwise Transparent file format whose markup, or absence of markup, has been arranged to thwart or discourage subsequent modification by readers is not Transparent. An image format is not Transparent if used for any substantial amount of text. A copy that is not "Transparent" is called "Opaque". Examples of suitable formats for Transparent copies include plain ASCII without markup, Texinfo input format, LaTeX input format, SGML or XML using a publicly available DTD, and standard-conforming simple HTML, PostScript or PDF designed for human modification. Examples of transparent image formats include PNG, XCF and JPG. Opaque formats include proprietary formats that can be read and edited only by proprietary word processors, SGML or XML for which the DTD and/or processing tools are not generally available, and the machine-generated HTML, PostScript or PDF produced by some word processors for output purposes only. The "Title Page" means, for a printed book, the title page itself, plus such following pages as are needed to hold, legibly, the material this License requires to appear in the title page. For works in formats which do not have any title page as such, "Title Page" means the text near the most prominent appearance of the work's title, preceding the beginning of the body of the text. A section "Entitled XYZ" means a named subunit of the Document whose title either is precisely XYZ or contains XYZ in parentheses following text that translates XYZ in another language. (Here XYZ stands for a specific section name mentioned below, such as "Acknowledgements", "Dedications", "Endorsements", or "History".) To "Preserve the Title" of such a section when you modify the Document means that it remains a section "Entitled XYZ" according to this definition. The Document may include Warranty Disclaimers next to the notice which states that this License applies to the Document. These Warranty Disclaimers are considered to be included by reference in this License, but only as regards disclaiming warranties: any other implication that these Warranty Disclaimers may have is void and has no effect on the meaning of this License.

2. VERBATIM COPYING

You may copy and distribute the Document in any medium, either commercially or noncommercially, provided that this License, the copyright notices, and the license notice saying this License applies to the Document are reproduced in all copies, and that you add no other conditions whatsoever to those of this License. You may not use technical measures to obstruct or control the reading or further copying of the copies you make or distribute. However, you may accept compensation in exchange for copies. If you distribute a large enough number of copies you must also follow the conditions in section 3. You may also lend copies, under the same conditions stated above, and you may publicly display copies.

3. COPYING IN QUANTITY

If you publish printed copies (or copies in media that commonly have printed covers) of the Document, numbering more than 100, and the Document's license notice requires Cover Texts, you must enclose the copies in covers that carry, clearly and legibly, all these Cover Texts: Front-Cover Texts on the front cover, and Back-Cover Texts on the back cover. Both covers must also clearly and legibly identify you as the publisher of these copies. The front cover must present the full title with all words of the title equally prominent and visible. You may add other material on the covers in addition. Copying with changes limited to the covers, as long as they preserve the title of the Document and satisfy these conditions, can be treated as verbatim copying in other respects. If the required texts for either cover are too voluminous to fit legibly, you should put the first ones listed (as many as fit reasonably) on the actual cover, and continue the rest onto adjacent pages. If you publish or distribute Opaque copies of the Document numbering more than 100, you must either include a machine-readable Transparent copy along with each Opaque copy, or state in or with each Opaque copy a computer-network location from which the general network-using public has access to download using public-standard network protocols a complete Transparent copy of the Document, free of added material. If you use the latter option, you must take reasonably prudent steps, when you begin distribution of Opaque copies in quantity, to ensure that this Transparent copy will remain thus accessible at the stated location until at least one year after the last time you distribute an Opaque copy (directly or through your agents or retailers) of that edition to the public. It is requested, but not required, that you contact the authors of the Document well before redistributing any large number of copies, to give them a chance to provide you with an updated version of the Document.

4. MODIFICATIONS

You may copy and distribute a Modified Version of the Document under the conditions of sections 2 and 3 above, provided that you release the Modified Version under precisely this License, with the Modified Version filling the role of the Document, thus licensing distribution and modification of the Modified Version to whoever possesses a copy of it. In addition, you must do these things in the Modified Version: A. Use in the Title Page (and on the covers, if any) a title distinct from that of the Document, and from those of previous versions (which should, if there were any, be listed in the History section of the Document). You may use the same title as a previous version if the original publisher of that version gives permission. B. List on the Title Page, as authors, one or more persons or entities responsible for authorship of the modifications in the Modified Version, together with at least five of the principal authors of the Document (all of its principal authors, if it has fewer than five), unless they release you from this requirement. C. State on the Title page the name of the publisher of the Modified Version, as the publisher. D. Preserve all the copyright notices of the Document. E. Add an appropriate copyright notice for your modifications adjacent to the other copyright notices. F. Include, immediately after the copyright notices, a license notice giving the public permission to use the Modified Version under the terms of this License, in the form shown in the Addendum below. G. Preserve in that license notice the full lists of Invariant Sections and required Cover Texts given in the Document's license notice. H. Include an unaltered copy of this License. I. Preserve the section Entitled "History", Preserve its Title, and add to it an item stating at least the title, year, new authors, and publisher of the Modified Version as given on the Title Page. If there is no section Entitled "History" in the Document, create one stating the title, year, authors, and publisher of the Document as given on its Title Page, then add an item describing the Modified Version as stated in the previous sentence. J. Preserve the network location, if any, given in the Document for public access to a Transparent copy of the Document, and likewise the network locations given in the Document for previous versions it was based on. These may be placed in the "History" section. You may omit a network location for a work that was published at least four years before the Document itself, or if the original publisher of the version it refers to gives permission. K. For any section Entitled "Acknowledgements" or "Dedications", Preserve the Title of the section, and preserve in the section all the substance and tone of each of the contributor acknowledgements and/or dedications given therein. L. Preserve all the Invariant Sections of the Document, unaltered in their text and in their titles. Section numbers or the equivalent are not considered part of the section titles. M. Delete any section Entitled "Endorsements". Such a section may not be included in the Modified Version. N. Do not retitle any existing section to be Entitled "Endorsements" or to conflict in title with any Invariant Section. O. Preserve any Warranty Disclaimers. If the Modified Version includes new front-matter sections or appendices that qualify as Secondary Sections and contain no material copied from the Document, you may at your option designate some or all of these sections as invariant. To do this, add their titles to the list of Invariant Sections in the Modified Version's license notice. These titles must be distinct from any other section titles. You may add a section Entitled "Endorsements", provided it contains nothing but endorsements of your Modified Version by various parties--for example, statements of peer review or that the text has been approved by an organization as the authoritative definition of a standard. You may add a passage of up to five words as a Front-Cover Text, and a passage of up to 25 words as a Back-Cover Text, to the end of the list of Cover Texts in the Modified Version. Only one passage of Front-Cover Text and one of Back-Cover Text may be added by (or through arrangements made by) any one entity. If the Document already includes a cover text for the same cover, previously added by you or by arrangement made by the same entity you are acting on behalf of, you may not add another; but you may replace the old one, on explicit permission from the previous publisher that added the old one. The author(s) and publisher(s) of the Document do not by this License give permission to use their names for publicity for or to assert or imply endorsement of any Modified Version.

5. COMBINING DOCUMENTS

You may combine the Document with other documents released under this License, under the terms defined in section 4 above for modified versions, provided that you include in the combination all of the Invariant Sections of all of the original documents, unmodified, and list them all as Invariant Sections of your combined work in its license notice, and that you preserve all their Warranty Disclaimers. The combined work need only contain one copy of this License, and multiple identical Invariant Sections may be replaced with a single copy. If there are multiple Invariant Sections with the same name but different contents, make the title of each such section unique by adding at the end of it, in parentheses, the name of the original author or publisher of that section if known, or else a unique number. Make the same adjustment to the section titles in the list of Invariant Sections in the license notice of the combined work. In the combination, you must combine any sections Entitled "History" in the various original documents, forming one section Entitled "History"; likewise combine any sections Entitled "Acknowledgements", and any sections Entitled "Dedications". You must delete all sections Entitled "Endorsements".

6. COLLECTIONS OF DOCUMENTS

You may make a collection consisting of the Document and other documents released under this License, and replace the individual copies of this License in the various documents with a single copy that is included in the collection, provided that you follow the rules of this License for verbatim copying of each of the documents in all other respects. You may extract a single document from such a collection, and distribute it individually under this License, provided you insert a copy of this License into the extracted document, and follow this License in all other respects regarding verbatim copying of that document.

7. AGGREGATION WITH INDEPENDENT WORKS

A compilation of the Document or its derivatives with other separate and independent documents or works, in or on a volume of a storage or distribution medium, is called an "aggregate" if the copyright resulting from the compilation is not used to limit the legal rights of the compilation's users beyond what the individual works permit. When the Document is included in an aggregate, this License does not apply to the other works in the aggregate which are not themselves derivative works of the Document. If the Cover Text requirement of section 3 is applicable to these copies of the Document, then if the Document is less than one half of the entire aggregate, the Document's Cover Texts may be placed on covers that bracket the Document within the aggregate, or the electronic equivalent of covers if the Document is in electronic form. Otherwise they must appear on printed covers that bracket the whole aggregate.

8. TRANSLATION

Translation is considered a kind of modification, so you may distribute translations of the Document under the terms of section 4. Replacing Invariant Sections with translations requires special permission from their copyright holders, but you may include translations of some or all Invariant Sections in addition to the original versions of these Invariant Sections. You may include a translation of this License, and all the license notices in the Document, and any Warranty Disclaimers, provided that you also include the original English version of this License and the original versions of those notices and disclaimers. In case of a disagreement between the translation and the original version of this License or a notice or disclaimer, the original version will prevail. If a section in the Document is Entitled "Acknowledgements", "Dedications", or "History", the requirement (section 4) to Preserve its Title (section 1) will typically require changing the actual title.

9. TERMINATION

You may not copy, modify, sublicense, or distribute the Document except as expressly provided for under this License. Any other attempt to copy, modify, sublicense or distribute the Document is void, and will automatically terminate your rights under this License. However, parties who have received copies, or rights, from you under this License will not have their licenses terminated so long as such parties remain in full compliance.

10. FUTURE REVISIONS OF THIS LICENSE

The Free Software Foundation may publish new, revised versions of the GNU Free Documentation License from time to time. Such new versions will be similar in spirit to the present version, but may differ in detail to address new problems or concerns. See http://www.gnu.org/copyleft/. Each version of the License is given a distinguishing version number. If the Document specifies that a particular numbered version of this License "or any later version" applies to it, you have the option of following the terms and conditions either of that specified version or of any later version that has been published (not as a draft) by the Free Software Foundation. If the Document does not specify a version number of this License, you may choose any version ever published (not as a draft) by the Free Software Foundation. ADDENDUM: How to use this License for your documents To use this License in a document you have written, include a copy of the License in the document and put the following copyright and license notices just after the title page: Copyright (c) YEAR YOUR NAME. Permission is granted to copy, distribute and/or modify this document under the terms of the GNU Free Documentation License, Version 1.2 or any later version published by the Free Software Foundation; with no Invariant Sections, no Front-Cover Texts, and no Back-Cover Texts. A copy of the license is included in the section entitled "GNU Free Documentation License". If you have Invariant Sections, Front-Cover Texts and Back-Cover Texts, replace the "with...Texts." line with this: with the Invariant Sections being LIST THEIR TITLES, with the Front-Cover Texts being LIST, and with the Back-Cover Texts being LIST. If you have Invariant Sections without Cover Texts, or some other combination of the three, merge those two alternatives to suit the situation. If your document contains nontrivial examples of program code, we recommend releasing these examples in parallel under your choice of free software license, such as the GNU General Public License, to permit their use in free software.

MIX
Papier aus verantwortungsvollen Quellen
Paper from responsible sources
FSC® C105338

Printed by Books on Demand GmbH, Norderstedt / Germany